# The Pride Guide

# The Pride Guide

## A Guide to Sexual and Social Health for LGBTQ Youth

Jo Langford

*Rowman & Littlefield*
Lanham • Boulder • New York • London

Published by Rowman & Littlefield
A wholly owned subsidiary of The Rowman & Littlefield Publishing Group, Inc.
4501 Forbes Boulevard, Suite 200, Lanham, Maryland 20706
www.rowman.com

Unit A, Whitacre Mews, 26-34 Stannary Street, London SE11 4AB

British Library Cataloguing in Publication Information Available

**Library of Congress Cataloging-in-Publication Data Is Available**

ISBN 978-1-5381-1076-8 (cloth: alk. paper)
ISBN 978-1-5381-1077-5 (electronic)

∞™ The paper used in this publication meets the minimum requirements of American National Standard for Information Sciences—Permanence of Paper for Printed Library Materials, ANSI/NISO Z39.48-1992.

Printed in the United States of America

# CONTENTS

CONTENTS

# ACKNOWLEDGMENTS

Thank you to the young queer people reading this; your efforts and energy are going to build on the evolutionary and cultural gains we have already made, and bring us into a deeper understanding of what gender, sex, and ultimately humanity mean.

Thank you to the parents and other grown-ups in the lives of our young queer folk. There are too many LGBT youth who are orphaned in this day and age—both physically and emotionally—and we have lost too many of these young people to shame, suicide, and the specific dangers of living on the street.

For my three most-importants, Amber, Xander, and 'Bella: You have taught me what it means to be strong, self-aware, and as much myself as I can be. I feel so fortunate that I am close to the man I always wanted to be. I am indebted to the three of you in more ways than I have words.

Thanks, also, to so many others who have been there for me: my family, friends (who also happen to be family), and colleagues (who also happen to be friends). Thank you all for the support, inspiration, conversation, patience, flames under my butt—and always, the palpable, palpable love.

And a very special thanks to my smart and enthusiastic focus group of LGBTQ people, professionals, and allies for the fantastic feedback and, ultimately, the endorsements! Your help, time, and opinions were integral to this resource.

# INTRO

I am a therapist, a sex educator, and a dad. I've worked for decades to bring information (with humor) to queer underagers to increase their knowledge and self-confidence. I see this as an essential, proactive defense against the sometimes-serious consequences that can accompany sexual activity, as well as the often-serious consequences of simply being queer in the world.

This book can help you protect lesbian, gay, bisexual, and transgender youth from some of the other trauma that can be associated with being both a teen and queer at the same time.

If you are a teenager, consider this:

- Approximately half of you are already sexually active in some way.[1]

- A quarter of you have already gotten a sexually transmitted infection (STI).[2]

- A third of you have received an aggressive solicitation from an online predator in the past year.[3]

- One out of every three of you has sent a nude picture to someone with your cell phone.[4]

- About one-third of you will have been sexually assaulted in some way before your eighteenth birthday.[5]

If you *also* happen to identify as G, L, B, T, or Q,

- At least one in ten of you has missed school in the last month because you did not feel safe.

- Approximately a third of you have been bullied at school (34 percent) or online (28 percent).

- You are twice as likely as your straight/cis counterparts to experience physical dating violence (18 percent vs. 8 percent).

- 40 percent of you have seriously considered suicide.

- As many as 30 percent of you have tried.[6]

This book will help you deal with people who will try to victimize you. Though you are stronger than others due to your struggles, more creative due to having to think outside larger, cultural boxes, and braver in the face of both external adversity and your own, unique, inner journey—you will *still* face adversity, invisibility, and violence, just because you are you. Predators and haters are real, as are the problems and barriers they will create for you, and we will talk about them throughout this book.

It is also common, now, for adolescent girls and boys (of all genders, orientations, and identities) to accidentally become their own worst enemy—especially where technology intersects with their sexuality. Much of the sexual damage being done to you, as individuals and as a generation, is being done to yourselves and each other.

## LGBTW

Peppered throughout the following chapters are smaller, "sidebar" bits of information that some readers will find relevant, titled LGBTW—a compound word mixing the LGBT initialism with the Internet shorthand BTW (for "by the way"). These time-out-of-time subsections are meant to expand on topics within the chapters or, in some cases, to add in an extra layer of consideration.

## LGBTW . . . The Values Contributing to This Work

I am a kinda crunchy, sorta groovy, West Coast, American, liberal, educated, secular, cisgender, bisexual, white dude. I am the dad of two amazing children, as well as a veteran sex educator, with decades of experience helping teenagers grapple with the many fun, fascinating, and sometimes frightening aspects of sex and sexuality. As such, I have a deep appreciation for the difficulty and confusion associated with puberty and adolescence—including having to navigate the wide landscape of both sexuality and gender.

My goal in writing this book is to share what I have learned from decades of working with young people, both boys and girls, both queer and straight, both trans and cis, and to be as helpful, inclusive, thorough, and empowering as possible.

As a person, a parent, *and* a professional,

- I believe teens ought to be held responsible for their own learning and experience, actions, and reactions.

- To achieve this, I believe they need to be treated with respect, have access to accurate and relevant comprehensive sexual education, and be held to high standards.

- I believe it is the responsibility of caring adults in young people's lives to provide such information and standards and to model the importance of acknowledging and accepting all sex orientations and gender identities.

- I believe that there are both risks and rewards inherent in sexual behavior, self-expression, and simply existing in the world as a queer person.

- I believe that fear and ignorance, vagueness, and avoidance increase those risks, and that frank, honest, medically accurate, and open-minded approaches lower them.

And I have written the following book with these values in mind.

## LGBTW . . . For Parents

This book is the product of decades of experience as a professional sex educator. The pages that follow contain straightforward, open discussions and descriptions of the critical issues surrounding sex, gender, and sexuality and expression that today's GLBT teenagers confront. I stand with the vast majority of child development and behavior experts—and decades of proven research that clear, complete information and education are our children's single most effective defense against the risks and dangers surrounding life as a queer teen—including sex, socialization, and societal attitudes, from low-level to life-threatening.

That said, you know your child best. For some teens, especially those thirteen and older, it may work best to simply give them this book and offer to discuss any questions that come up. For younger tweens, I recommend that you read this book first and consider using it as a guide for discussion.

The final section of this book, Part Ten, is written specifically for parents and other supportive adults in the lives of young LGBTQ people.

## LGBTW . . . For Readers

Same-sex attraction, non-binary gender, and people not conforming to cultural expectations of their biological sex or perceived gender are not recent developments. Most countries and cultures have a recorded history of people whose behavior and identity fall into the categories we now call bisexuality, homosexuality, transgender, intersex, asexuality, etc.

North and South American tribal traditions and rituals. Australian aboriginals. Greek gods. Queens and kings. Scientists and philosophers. Performers and artists. The world would not be what it was if not for the influence of notable figures in the development of GLBT history and culture,[7,8,9] such as Leonardo da Vinci, Oscar Wilde, Gertrude Stein, Alan Turing, First Lady Eleanor Roosevelt, Harvey Milk, Dan Parent, Ryan Murphy, and RuPaul.

Though there is much confusion, panic, conflict, and violence in the world now, it is important to remember and honor not only the brave and unapologetic people who have paved roads and started conversations, but to honor the brave and unapologetic in yourself as well.

What will you contribute?

## My Big List of Disclaimers

This book is intended to provide information, education, and inspiration. It is intended to be an adjunct to—not a substitute for—professional, medical, or legal advice. Laws and practices vary state-by-state, region-by-region, country-by-country. In addition, much of the information included here can and (most likely) will change with time and with the rapid development of technology, science, and culture. It is in your best interest to confirm any content inside (and its relevance to your own life and circumstance) by doing your own research.

This writing is a snapshot in time (and at a time when we are *all* learning new things about these dynamics). Though I believe I have done due diligence in terms of gathering both information and feedback (and will continue to seek and welcome feedback for future editions), I am sure there are topics and targets I have missed. I hope that any and all feedback will be given with the same optimism, helpful intent, and open spirit with which I give you this book. As twenty-first-century poet Zac Efron once said, "We're all in this together."

### LGBTW . . . Intent

My goal in writing this book is to share what I know from decades of working with young people, both boys and girls, both queer and straight, both trans and cis, and to be as inclusive, thorough, and empowering as possible. The language and emphasis used throughout this book is intended in a very deep and genuine way to be helpful (not hateful), inclusive (not alienating), thorough (not marginalizing), and empowering (not offensive). This writer wholly supports non-binary concepts, the use of inclusive language, and the right for everyone to determine what their bodies mean to them. That being said, for the purposes of this book, this writer does occasionally use phrases such as, "born in a female body," "natal/biological male," "gendered female at birth," and "female reproductive system." This language is used alongside more open and inclusive language and primarily limited to the chapters and sections referring to specific biological processes (and in places in which I struggled to create openness without sacrificing detail). The use of these phrases is not meant to be arbitrary, limiting, contributing to any gender-based oppression, or disrespectful to anyone, and I hope that it is not taken as such.

## LGBTW . . . Pronouns

This writer supports the individual choice of pronouns, and uses the singular, "they," and its derivatives (them, their, etc.) throughout this book in an attempt at inclusion. For more information about the pronoun and the rationale behind its use, see chapter 7.

## LGBTW . . . Genetics and Generalizations

Humans typically have forty-six chromosomes that contain our DNA—our unique "code" that tells our cells how to perform. Twenty-three of our chromosomes came from a sperm cell and twenty-three came from an egg. Those two sets of twenty-three cells make up our forty-six chromosomes. Some pairs determine eye color, some determine how sensitive our skin is, and two of them (called X and Y—presumably because of their shape under microscopes) are the sex chromosomes. This pair determines if you are born male ("XY") or born female ("XX").[10]

Of course there are exceptions in terms of the miracle-that-is-human-biology, *and* there are other variations on occasion, but most people are XY or XX.

Most people, however, do not know their sex (on a genetic level) for sure. There are tests (called karyotyping) that can check, but unless your mother had a test called amniocentesis while she was pregnant with you, you may not have certainty about your XX or XY status—most babies are assigned male or female at birth, based on the presence of either a penis or vagina when they were born.

It's important to acknowledge that this is the norm, that there are always exceptions (XXX, XXY, XYY are examples), *and* for the purposes of *this* book, terminology such as "natal male," "assigned female at birth," "born a boy," or "born with a female body" may be used to refer to people who were designated "male" or "female" based on the external genitals with which they were born.

Acknowledging that there is some semantic debate about phrases such as "female genitals" and "boy parts," this writer believes that biological sex and gender identity are connected, though not the same.

Gender identity is not created at birth the way sexual identity is. Gender identity is also not created externally, by someone else the way one's sex is—gender identity is sorted and developed with time and experience in relation and reaction to one's sex. It's an internal development that primarily comes from within each person.

Some people born with typically male chromosomal patterns or genitalia grow to identify as men/male. Some do not. Some people born with typically female genetic markers or genitalia grow to identify as women/female. Others do not.

Someone can be born in a particular state, say, California. That is an *external*, factual, and situational designation that people are assigning that child: "Californian." Now that child through the course of their life may or may not remain in California and could relocate to perhaps, New York—another factual and situational designation, making them (by definition) now a "New Yorker."

This person's identity can be completely separate from the physical state they live in. Yes, they may move through their physical community and even pay taxes as a "Californian" or a "New Yorker" (and perhaps there was even that summer after college when they briefly tried out being a "Texan" with their roommate), but the way in which they identify might be different. They may completely adopt the "New Yorker" identity once they physically live in New York for a period of time. They may also identify as a "Californian," through and through, despite living on the East Coast for several years. These things are related, but separate—like gender identity developed through experience and sexual identity assigned at birth.

This writer does not believe that the current social problems associated with ignorance, misunderstandings, hatred, and transphobia are about the sex assignations and descriptions associated with bodies at birth, but with cultural difficulties around being inflexible about how those descriptors relate to the development of a particular person's gender identity.

To hold that someone born in California must identify, forever and always, as Californian despite their geographical and philosophical changes and internal experience, is misguided and kind of stupid. In fact, just as there can be massive differences between areas such as Manhattan and Upstate New York (though both are *in* New York) or even closer areas such as L.A. and "The Valley" (*super* different, though both technically Los Angeles), components of biological sex—chromosomes, genitals, hormones—exist on a spectrum as well.

To be clear, components of sex and gender are more complex than simply external genitalia, *and* components of sex and gender are connected but separate. In fact, all components of sex from genitals to hormones to chromosomes exist on a spectrum rather than as a binary.

We now know that gender does not simply exist in a polarized way, either "boy" or "girl"—it is a spectrum in which most everyone with human parts expresses and identifies with different aspects of both masculinity and femininity.

So as you read this, keep in mind that though the sex of a body may be assigned (generally within a binary) at birth by others, the gender identity of a person is created by how aligned (or not) that person feels in said body.

This book will help you to become your own best advocate by helping you prioritize your health and safety, increase your level of self-care and personal responsibility, and make choices about your sexuality and gender expression that will work for you.

This book also offers a safe, private way to obtain the skills and information you need to make informed decisions, *and* it will give you the crucial tools with which to approach sex and sexuality with a sense of confidence and seriousness, having fun along the way while doing as little harm to yourselves and each other as possible.

## PART ONE
# "BORN THIS WAY"

Having a clear understanding of the human body (yours as well as others') is a huge part of successfully navigating puberty, a healthy, adult sexual life, and even old age. Some body parts are reproductive, some are sexual, and some are both. Some people are born with certain parts, others are not, and some lose or acquire them later through surgery, hormones, or other medical interventions.

# BIOLOGY

Not everyone with **female sexual and reproductive body parts** identifies as a female, though most people gendered as female at birth have anatomical similarities.

The **vagina,** for example, is the main reproductive organ for female animals. It can also be called the birth canal, and it is close to (but separate from) the urethra (where the pee comes out of the body). The vagina has numerous nicknames including "gyne" (pronounced "jine") or, sometimes the slightly more crass "pussy," and is the primary pathway both for sperm to reach the cervix and eventually the fallopian tubes (so pregnancy can begin), and for a baby to leave the uterus (when pregnancy ends). Vaginas also pass blood and substances during menstruation and can self-lubricate in preparation for sex.

Within the vagina is the **cervix**—the small, mini-doughnut-shaped organ that serves as a gateway between the uterus and the back of the vagina. **The Gräfenberg spot**, or "G-spot," is also contained within the vagina. The G-spot is a small area of tissues typically found behind the pubic bone on the inner, front wall of the vagina (toward the belly button). Many people report that when massaged or stimulated, the G-spot can become swollen, feel quite pleasurable, and can contribute to powerful sexual feelings including orgasm. The G-spot has a reputation of being unique, elusive, and mysterious to some people. It is possible that some people may not have a G-spot, probable that others may have difficulty locating theirs (or others'), and certain that each person develops their own relationship to their G-spot when/if they do.

The part of the female reproductive system that is visible on the outside is referred to as the **vulva.** Though some refer to this generally as a vagina, technically the vagina is on the inside. Above the pubic bone, and under the belly button is the **mons**—the part where the pubic hair grows. Below that are two sets of labia (or lips): the **labia minora** (the inner ones) protect the vagina and are protected themselves by the **labia majora** (the outer ones).

Near the top of the labia is a short protrusion with a very, very sensitive tip called the **clitoris**. The clitoris is covered with a small fold of skin (called the clitoral hood), and has no other function other than pleasure, as it contains a massive amount of nerve endings packed into a very small space. It is located above the urethra, at the top of the opening of the vagina, and is an important part of sexual pleasure for the people who have one.

The **uterus** is located behind the cervix of the vagina. This is the womb where an embryo could attach itself and eventually grow into a fetus during pregnancy if an egg becomes fertilized in the fallopian tubes. The **fallopian tubes** are a 7- to 14-centimeter-long pathway connecting the uterus to the **ovaries**, where eggs are produced, stored, and from where they are released during ovulation.

Eggs contain the female DNA and twenty-three chromosomes, which, if joined by the chromosomes and male DNA of a sperm, create an embryo.

Not everyone with **male sexual and reproductive body parts** identifies as a male, though most people gendered a male at birth have anatomical similarities.

For example, the **penis** is the primary reproductive organ for male creatures. The penis has numerous nicknames including "dick" or sometimes the slightly more crass "cock," and is the main delivery method of sperm when it exits the body during ejaculation. Different than the vagina, it also contains the urethra, and also serves as the male method of urination.

The sac of skin and muscle that contains and protects the **testicles** is called the **scrotum**, and is located between the anus and the penis. The testicles themselves are balls of approximately 850 feet of tube and other materials that make the male hormone testosterone, and produce sperm. Commonly called "balls," they come in all kinds of sizes, but are generally round and typically come as a pair.

The **sperm** produced by the testicles are the main, male reproductive cells and contain the male DNA and twenty-three chromosomes. Sperm are stored in a second layer of tubes collected at the top of each testicle, called the **epididymis**, where they can grow and mature. If sperm is joined with the chromosomes and female DNA of an egg, an embryo is created.

Some people with penises have a double-layered fold of skin called a **foreskin**. Sometimes this extra skin is removed (for different reasons) during a surgery called circumcision. This painful and sometimes controversial surgery is most popular in some religious traditions and typically done within a few days or weeks of a baby's birth.

For uncircumcised people, the foreskin protects the sensitive head (or the **glans**) of the penis when it is not erect, and retracts when they are aroused and their penis becomes erect. If a person is circumcised, their glans is always exposed.

Circumcision is relatively rare worldwide (approximately 16 percent in Britain[1]), and has been declining in popularity over the last several decades in the United States and Canada. According to the Centers for Disease Control and Prevention (CDC), only around half of all male-gendered babies released from American hospitals still have their foreskins removed, which means that if you become sexually active with someone with a penis, there is almost a 50/50 chance that their penis will be uncircumcised.

An erect penis is also called an "erection," a "hard on," a "boner," and probably literally a million other terms, and forms a clear pathway for sperm to leave the body during ejaculation. Urine also leaves the body this way, but most people with penises find peeing while having an erection . . . let's call it problematic.

During arousal, sperm stored in the epididymis leave the testicles via tubes called the **vas deferens**, picking up fluids from other glands along the way. The fluids eventually form a milky substance called semen that protects the sperm and helps them travel to their next destination.

One of those glands encountered along their journey is called the **prostate gland**. The prostate is jokingly (though accurately) called the "male G-spot." It is located a couple of inches inside the anus and forward along the front wall of the rectum (toward the belly button). Like the G-spot, stimulation of the prostate gland, through massage, can feel very pleasurable to some people.

# PUBERTY

**P**uberty is the process that signals the start of adolescence, when your child body begins to change into your adult body. It's the transition between childhood and adulthood.

Both male and female bodies will begin to take on different characteristics and shapes during the process of puberty. The speed and timing for this can be different—anywhere from one to six years. But regardless of the timeline, for everyone, puberty comes with new thoughts and feelings as hormones trigger both physical and emotional changes.

Medical professionals are able to prescribe puberty blockers to hit the pause button on puberty for trans children, buying them some time to make plans and choices, and find resources and support. In the absence of prescribed puberty blockers, puberty in female bodies usually begins between the ages of eight and thirteen; for male bodies it's usually between the ages of nine and fourteen.[1] Whether encouraged or slowed by medical treatments or left to progress on its own, the age at which the process of puberty starts can be different for everyone, but we all end up in our adult bodies eventually.

When puberty starts, the brain releases chemicals called hormones, which are responsible for all of the physical changes in our bodies. In natal girls, these hormones stimulate the ovaries to produce hormones called estrogen and progesterone. In natal boys, they stimulate the testicles to produce testosterone.

Other hormones trigger bodies to develop in other ways as well. Muscles, bones, external limbs, and internal organs shift to change our overall body shape. One of the earliest signs of puberty for both sexes is hair growth. Hair grows under arms, on legs, and around genitals, and may show up in a couple of other random places as well. Hair becomes thicker as puberty progresses.

Typically between the ages of twelve and sixteen,[2] natal boys will experience muscle growth development in their external genitals and begin growing hair in various places on their body, including their chest, face, and pubic area. They will begin to develop sperm and may experience spontaneous erections.

Typically between the ages of ten and twelve, the bodies of natal girls usually become curvier with hip and breast development; hair growth begins as well, overall body fat increases, and menstrual periods can start.[3]

The timing, intensity, and duration of puberty are affected by genetic factors (your body's shape and size, and your family history, etc.) and environmental factors (nutrition, exercise, stress level, etc.). During this time, it is important to develop a healthy relationship to your own body, and basic hygiene behaviors are a great place to begin.

**Hygiene** refers to the (probably-should-be-daily) routines and rituals we use to keep our bodies clean and healthy. For most people, basic hygiene includes their body, teeth, clothes, and some kind of effort with their hair. Some level of attention paid to finger- and toenails, choosing whether or not to use a body scent or hair product, dealing with acne and body odor, and deciding whether or not to shave your underarms, face, legs (and maybe other parts) are also part of personal hygiene.

**Body odor** is created when bacteria and sweat in certain body areas—specifically underarms, hair, and feet—become fragrant. Body odor (or "B.O.") is natural for everyone, but it can be more intense for teens. All humans have smells, many of which are pleasant and make us unique and attractive to others, and some of which do not. In adolescence, hormones can turn up the volume of those natural fragrances. It's your choice whether to let your fragrances run wild, to balance them out with other fragrances, or to mask them by showering in body spray (which can also be problematic). Whatever your choice, do it on purpose. Bathing regularly and carrying "emergency" deodorant with you for touch-ups can help you choose and control the amount of personal scent you share with others.

**Acne** is also triggered by hormones during puberty. These are minor infections, called pimples (or zits), caused by skin pores becoming clogged with oil and dirt. Squeezing them will only make them angry and cause the infection to spread.

The simplest way to keep your pores clean is to wash your skin regularly and thoroughly with a cleansing product—not necessarily soap, which can dry out your skin, causing it to produce more oils in response. If you're concerned about your acne, it is worth visiting your doctor or a dermatologist for an expert opinion (and possibly, a prescription skin cream, gel, or lotion), but remembering to rinse your face with warm water and drying it off with a clean towel a handful of times each day is enough for many people to keep the "good' oils your skin needs, while cleaning off the excess and/or "bad" oils that clog pores.

Other things that can help include keeping a balanced diet, keeping your hands and hair away from your face, and keeping your sheets and pillowcases clean. Bathing or showering before going to bed (rather than when you wake up in the morning) can help achieve this.

## LGBTW . . . Pubic Hair

Pubic hair is the hair that grows on and around your genitals. Everyone's genitals can be unique, but we all have pubic hair. This hair can be thicker and curlier than the hair on your head. You may find it annoying or distracting, or you may not have ever given it a lick of thought, but it is actually kind of important.

Pubic hair provides a protective shield against certain kinds of bacteria and provides a bit of cushioning against the grinding friction of sexual activity. Pubic hair also holds natural body scents that other people's brains can interpret as sexy, and is a signal that your body is developing into its adult form.

Some people let their pubic hair do whatever it decides to do, while others feel the urge to style it (much as people do the hair on their heads). Some people do light grooming with scissors or clippers, others trim bonsai-like shapes into their pubic hair, and some blade-shave it completely.

The problem with shaving your pubic area is that it can leave microscopic open wounds, and in warm, dark environments—which your crotch probably is, most of the time—that skin can become irritated, inflamed, and become a home for not-so-great bacteria. Shaving your swimsuit area completely also leaves you vulnerable to certain STIs (like herpes), can be super itchy, and can sting like you've been attacked by something.

Nature puts pubic hair there for a reason, and there is absolutely no reason anyone should feel weird or self-conscious about it. If you feel that you must do some landscaping below your belt, try to limit it to trimming the hedges a bit rather than mowing the whole damn lawn.

# IF YOU WERE BORN WITH FEMALE REPRODUCTIVE PARTS

**M**enstruation (also called a "period") is considered the beginning of someone's menstrual cycle—a fairly involved physical and emotional cycle that is the female reproductive system's way of preparing for a potential pregnancy.

Most people born with a female reproductive system, regardless of their gender or sexual identity, go through a process of discharging the material (including blood) that could have formed a nourishing home in their uterus for an embryo to grow into a fetus. If that person's body does not become pregnant, that unused material is released through their vaginal canal. This process typically repeats about once a month—cycles typically last twenty-eight days, but can vary from person to person.

The actual bleeding part is called the menstrual phase, and can last from two to seven days, depending on the person. The substance released (sometimes called a flow) is more than just blood. It contains other fluids, tissues, and unneeded and unused material, and can be inconsistent in its timing, duration, color, and amount.

Midway through a person's menstrual cycle, hormones trigger ovaries to release an egg. This is the proliferative phase of the cycle, more commonly called ovulation. The egg begins to journey through the fallopian tubes, reaching the uterus two to three days later. If that egg were to encounter and/or be fertilized by sperm, resulting in a pregnancy, it would typically happen during this time.

Because of this, people going through menstruation are considered most likely to get pregnant between day ten and day eighteen of their menstrual cycle. This is called the luteal or secretory phase and involves the lining of the uterus thickening with nutrients to make it possible for any fertilized eggs that might show up to implant and begin growing into a baby.

If this doesn't happen—no fertilization, no embryo, no baby—the uterus "reboots" itself, flushing out the thickened lining and nutrients (called the endrometrium), the actual period substance, and another cycle begins. . . .

Typically, first periods occur around age twelve or thirteen. However, some people can begin having periods as young as eight years old, and others may not start until they're sixteen.[1] Of course, if you are trans or on any kind of puberty blockers, this may be different for you. Once menstruation begins, it continues until menopause occurs, around the age of fifty, when monthly menstrual cycles change and eventually end.

The word *period* is one euphemism for the period of time when a girl is actively bleeding, and a non-offensive term most people use. Other terms people use are loaded with shame and embarrassment, and some are nicknames that families have adopted to help make conversations around it less awkward.

Here's a list that people have shared with me, which can help bring a little humor and empowerment to the process[2]:

- Aunt Flo
- The Bleedies
- Code red
- Cousin from the south
- The dot
- Girly flu
- Leak week
- Little visitor
- Monthlies
- On the dot (or on the rag)
- Red week

- Special time

- Surfing the crimson wave

- That time of the month

- Wetting the rag

A period can help some people feel like they are connected to their body and/or that they are growing up. For others, it may feel unsettling, awkward, or that they are not in control of their own development. Regardless of how you identify, there is no shame in having the hormones and body parts that make your monthly cycle possible.

Most people release only a few ounces of period fluid each day, and there are numerous methods people can use to manage that flow. These methods have been (unfortunately and somewhat controversially) called feminine hygiene products, but that term is limited, alienating, and rife with cultural ick. Call them whatever you'd like, but this writer favors terms that are more factual and inclusive and less judgy, like "menstrual products" or "period care products." You could also skip the generalized term once you find a favorite and just refer to your product by its brand name.

No matter your budget or lifestyle, you can find a method that can work for you. If you have just started menstruating or are prone to heavier flows, then pads may be a good choice. Size, eco-friendliness, comfort, and absorbency can all vary by brand. Generally, pads are flat, absorbent strips, with a blend of natural and synthetic fibers on one side, and a strip of adhesive on the other side to anchor it to your underwear and keep it in place. Pads collect period discharge throughout the day (and can be super effective while sleeping) and are discarded and replaced as needed.

Tampons are tiny, absorbent pods composed primarily of cotton, and/or other natural and synthetic fibers, which are inserted into the vagina during a period. As with pads, the size, absorbency, and method of insertion can vary, but many people report that tampons are more convenient than pads, and can be a comfortable choice for more experienced and/or active people.

A third popular option is the menstrual cup—a flexible, silicon, bell-shaped thimble, which can be inserted into the vagina to catch the period substances and then emptied and reinserted.

Regardless of the method that works best for you (and there are more than what are listed here), best practices for menstrual products include keeping a stock handy, and following the recommended schedule for changing them. When left in too long, bacteria can build up, releasing toxins into the body and potentially leading to an illness called toxic shock syndrome, which (though rare) can cause fevers, headaches, rashes, and irritation and eventually seizures.[3]

Accidents, leaks, and stains can happen during a period. These can be ill-timed, annoying, and embarrassing, but getting familiar with your cyclic patterns can help lower the number of surprises. Having spare products and a change of clothes in the trunk of your car, or your locker, can help in case of leaks, and hydrogen peroxide, salt, or baking soda should take care of most stains.

Despite the presence of blood, there is no actual wound, although many people on their period experience muscle pain, cramping, and discomfort. This can often be worse during adolescence. Your period also will not just flow freely out of you, as it would with an actual wound. Most people can discharge between four and twelve tablespoons each cycle,[4] spread out over two to seven days during each cycle.

Periods can be mysterious and misunderstood, and they have been shrouded in myth for generations. Some of the most popular ones include:

- **You can't have sex during your period.** Though some people choose not to, some people do.

- **You can't get pregnant if you have sex during your period.** Periods *and* sperm can last up to five days and some girls' cycles are shorter than others . . . you do the math. (But use protection while you do.)

- **If you don't have a period, that means you are pregnant.** Many things can contribute to missed, irregular, or nonexistent periods including weight, health issues, stress, nutrition, and hormonal changes from age, contraception, or hormone replacement therapy.

- **You can control the flow of your period, holding it in like you can with urine.** Um, no.

- **Sharks and bears will attack you if you are menstruating.**
  Again, no.

Some people have cycles that are "regular"—always roughly the same length, and about the same flow—and some do not. Either way, it can be helpful to keep track of your cycle. Tracking your cycle with an app or a calendar can help you note which days you may be most fertile (able to get pregnant), keep an eye out for any concerning changes (such as a missed period), and proactively prepare for the emotional and physical effects that some people experience during their period.

Those effects are called PMS (for premenstrual syndrome) or PMT (premenstrual tension), and can include a range of symptoms. Most people who have periods (approximately 85 percent[5] of them) experience some discomfort during the time between ovulation and menstruation. These symptoms are usually predictable, and can worsen the closer you get to your period—that's the "pre" part.

Some people report mood swings and emotions ranging from depression and sadness to crankiness and irritability, and/or muscle cramps and physical pain in their abdomen, breasts, or head. Some people get sleepy, some gain weight, and some crave certain foods. Tracking your cycle can help you predict what (if any) PMS/PMT symptoms you may experience and prepare for them.

Things that can help[6]:

- A go-to "uniform" can be both comfortable and comforting.

- Mind your cravings. Sugar, salt, and caffeine (although they can sound like a great idea in the moment) can exacerbate some PMS/PMT symptoms, making symptoms such as fatigue, bloating, and headaches worse. Try to eat them sparingly; or better yet, stick to protein and fresh fruits and vegetables.

- Good chocolate containing 60 percent or more of cacao can improve your mood, reduce cravings and stress, and give you a dose of magnesium, which can help with cramping.

- Water.

- Water.

- Water.

- Exercise. Keeping your body moving (even if you feel like just lying on the floor) can release endorphins, which can improve your mood and provide a nice distraction.

- Pain relief. Ibuprofen or acetaminophen can reduce muscle soreness caused by cramping. So can having an orgasm (either with a partner or just by yourself).

- Heat. Heating pads, blankets, oversize mugs of tea, and even small animals to cuddle with can help keep your abdomen warm and soothed.

- Be nice to yourself. If lying around in a giant sweater with your hair in a ponytail, binge-watching mid-1990s teen dramas does it for you, then do it! A person can potentially spend the equivalent of six years of their life menstruating,[7] so if you are one of them—use your periods as time to do something nice for yourself.

---

### LGBTW . . . Douches

We are all constantly bombarded with ads and clickbait designed to make us feel inappropriately and unnecessarily body-conscious. One of the worst culprits is the concept of the vaginal douche. Genitals have natural odor, and most of the time these scents register in other people's brains as pleasurable, and contribute to attraction and other sexy feelings. Vaginas are no exception to this. Like any body odor, there can be an abyss in which a lack of hygiene or some other issue can contribute to a funkiness that can register in other people's brains as less-than-pleasurable. Vaginas are not immune to this either.

Decent and consistent hygiene should counterbalance any natural funk to which your body is prone. If you have a vagina and are concerned or uncomfortable with your own scents, a gynecologist can help. The manufacturers and advertisers of douche products encourage you to insert fragrances and other chemicals into your vagina to avoid that "not so fresh"

---

feeling. These products are almost always unnecessary, outdated, and were most popular in the 1950s.

Today, douches tend to be

- prescribed by professionals in only rare and specific circumstances,

- a sanitary choice some people make before anal sex, or

- those guys (they tend to be male-identified) who obviously and purposely think themselves too hip, too sexy, and (try) too much, stinking up the room with faux and forced charm, pseudo-macho selfishness, and self-promotion.

OK, back to vaginas. . . . Douching can upset the ecosystem of a healthy vagina, and raise that vagina-haver's risk for a number of health issues, including cancer and some sexually transmitted infections.[8] In general, unless prescribed by a doctor, there is no reason you should need to douche your vagina.

**Breasts.** Western culture places a strange emphasis on breasts; their shapes, sizes, and mixed messages are rampant. You can be treated differently if you have particularly large or especially small breasts (also known as "boobs" or the more crass "tits"). Large breasts are painful and awkward to deal with, and they can also come with the weight of constant attention and negative judgment. Some people with smaller breasts may feel inadequate. Breast implants make some women feel more attractive, but such implants also shorten their life spans—and make them statistically three times more likely to kill themselves.[9] People with breasts can be inundated with judgment both by people who don't have any and by others that do, and with idealized or unrealistic standards about breast size.

Being as comfortable with your own body as you can, taking care of your body, and keeping your body as healthy as possible is your job as you navigate your own, unique pubescence. In doing so, it is possible to rise above the expectations and judgments of others. Your own self-esteem and risk for breast cancer may be less obvious than what is under your shirt, but they are infinitely more important than the size of your breasts.

While we are on the topic, *anyone* with breasts is at risk for breast cancer, regardless of your gender or how you self-identify. This is particularly true for cis women and trans men, though cis men can develop breast cancer as well, and (even after having surgery to remove their breasts) there may still be breast tissue that can develop cancer in trans men. Your risk is even greater if breast cancer runs in your family.

An x-ray mammogram of your breast at a doctor's office can help to detect cancer, though because 40 percent of diagnosed breast cancers are detected by people who feel a lump in their own breast,[10] Johns Hopkins Medical Center encourages monthly breast self-exams. Regularly examining your own breasts makes it more likely you will notice any changes in shape or texture that could signal the need for a professional examination.

Breast cancer affects millions of people, and early detection saves lives. There are loads of videos and resources online with guidelines on how to do this properly, and nationalbreastcancer.org/breast-self-exam is a great place to start. Don't freak out if you notice anything irregular—breasts can change with age and development, or during puberty or hormone replacement therapy (HRT). Statistically 80 percent of detected lumps are not cancerous, but you should make an appointment with your doctor[11] if you notice anything out of the ordinary.

**Gynecology** is the study of the female reproductive system. Medical professionals that specialize in this are called OB/GYNs, which is short for a doctor of obstetrics (pregnancy and childbirth) and/or gynecology (reproductive biology). It is a common—but completely untrue—belief that lesbians or trans men don't need gynecologic care. If you have any physical parts of the female reproductive system, it is important to see a gynecologist for regular check-ups. The American College of Obstetricians and Gynecologists recommends that anyone with female reproductive parts have their first visit with an OB/GYN (or similarly qualified professional) between the ages of thirteen and fifteen.[12] Your pediatrician may also be an option for you as long as you are legally a minor.

If you identify as trans, it is important to find a medical professional—if not an OB/GYN, then a family nurse practitioner or licensed midwife who specializes in trans health issues. The majority of doctors licensed and trained to administer hormones are also OB/GYNs. Until and unless you have a full hysterectomy, you will likely still need OB/GYN care and treatment in some capacity.

Periods for trans men are similar to those had by cis women; however, if you are taking hormones your period will stop, most likely within the first year, and birth control for most trans men becomes no longer necessary. If you are a trans guy and not on hormones, you will still have periods and can still get pregnant (depending on what kinds of sex you have), and even though you may no longer need birth control because your periods have stopped, that does not mean you do not still need to be using safer sex practices (see chapter 22).

When you become sexually active (whether with the same sex, opposite sex, or both), gynecologic care *and* STI counseling and testing become even more important.

You might feel a bit uncomfortable or embarrassed at the prospect of visiting your doctor, but it's super important for your sexual health—especially if you have a family history of reproductive health issues, are sexually active, or if you are pregnant.

Appointments usually involve a physical examination, similar to what you have had in the past, though the conversations about your body and health will become more detailed as you get older.

As you get further into puberty, your doctor will examine your breasts and external genitalia to screen for any concerns or changes as your body develops.

By the time you reach adulthood (or sooner if you become sexually active before that), your gynecological exams will also include an internal examination of your vagina. During this examination, your doctor will hold your vagina open with a tool called a speculum so they can feel your ovaries and uterus to check for any irregularities. They will also administer a pap smear, a swabbing of cells from your cervix, which they will use to test for human papillomavirus (HPV) and signs of cancer. These exams are generally not painful, but don't have a reputation of being very comfortable.

Some people choose to bring a support person to their appointments, especially in the beginning. As you get older, and your health care becomes more important, your privacy will become more important as well. Even if you have support people come with you, your doctor may ask them to give you privacy while you talk so that you can be as honest and open with your doctor as possible—even your parents. In fact, no one will make you have a parent in the room during doctor visits if you do not want that.

Conversations with your doctor are totally confidential, and it is OK to ask any questions and speak openly and honestly about your body, your sexual behavior, or any other issue. A doctor cannot legally share any of your personal information with anyone, including your parents, unless they have a reason to believe your life or your health is in danger.

---

### LGBTW . . . Insurance

Depending on whether or not you have health insurance (and, if you do, what your health care plan covers), access to a doctor may not be easy or even possible. Even if and when there is access, some of the specific medical treatments you may need may not be covered. This can be particularly difficult for trans men who may have already changed their gender marker to male, though are still in need of gynecologic care. Progressive health insurance policies and politics are in flux, and may not cover OB/GYN treatments for males. Your doctor should be able to help you navigate this, and find ways to get your health care needs met. If that is not possible for some reason, community-based clinics (such as Planned Parenthood) are the next logical step.

---

# IF YOU WERE BORN WITH MALE REPRODUCTIVE PARTS

The relationship that the average person with a penis has with their penis can be very powerful.

Though some trans folks can be indifferent about their penis, cis men (both gay and straight) can be quite obsessive about theirs—the sizes, the shapes, and the activity. They play with them their whole lives, they brag about them to others, and worry about them when alone.

Penises can be at once the brunt and source of a ridiculous amount of humor and an almost endless supply of insults:

- dork,
- dingus,
- tool,
- knob,
- goober,
- wienie,
- pecker,
- prick,
- dick,
- dickhead, and
- wanker

are all well-known insults based on penis euphemisms. Despite (or perhaps because of that), penises tend to be bragged about, protected vigilantly, and played with constantly. There are people with vaginas who may go their entire lives without ever taking the time to actually look at their vagina. But natal men start forming a relationship with their penis as soon as they discover it—some babies even find their penis in utero. And, even into adulthood, most people with penises fall asleep holding onto them like they're guarding them from thieves.

As with breasts, some people can get their self-esteem wrapped up with the size of their penis. This is called "boner shame." Despite all of the attention they get, penises can be confusing—even for people who have them—and most people do not have a realistic idea of how big the average penis is.

The only other erect penises most people see while growing up, besides their own, are in porn. The penises one sees in porn are not typically representative of the average penis (those guys are not in those movies because of their acting ability). Even the angles that the average person uses when they take a picture of their penis involve distorted perspectives.

P.S., stop doing that.

These distorted and unrealistic images can give some people the sense that their penis doesn't measure up . . . literally. The reality is that most penises are basically the same length when erect (hard), with the average penis measuring at approximately 5.6 inches when erect.[1] In fact, only five people out of every one hundred have an erection longer than six inches.[2]

Another confusing factor is that there are two different types of penises: "growers" and "showers." Growers are shorter when soft, but can double or even triple in length when hard. Showers, by comparison, remain approximately the same length whether flaccid or erect.

And on top of that, the size of a penis when it is soft (or flaccid) has nothing to do with its size when it is hard (or erect). This means that the 20 percent of the population that are growers and the 80 percent of the population that are showers all end up somewhere around 5.5 inches in the end.

The penis has two primary functions: releasing urine from the body (during urination) and releasing semen (during ejaculation). Both of these fluids are released through a long tube in the penis called the urethra, and neither of those functions has anything to do with its size. Along either side of the urethra are two, long, spongy tubes called the corpus cavernosa.

The process from erection to ejaculation has several steps involving your brain and the muscles, nerves, and blood vessels of the penis.

First the person becomes sexually aroused. Almost anything can cause arousal: sights, sounds, smells, touch, movement, memory, bouncy car rides, soft stuff. . . . These kinds of stimuli trigger the brain to send signals through the autonomic nervous system and spinal cord to the muscle fibers in the corpora cavernosa.[3]

The unique muscle fibers in the cavernosa then relax, allowing blood to enter (like blowing up one of those balloon-animal balloons, but using pressurized blood instead of pressurized air). Like fingers holding air in the balloon, muscles in the pelvic floor (called pubococcygeal muscles[4]) squeeze to keep the blood inside the cavernosa keeping the penis erect. These are the same muscles used to hold in urine when there isn't a restroom nearby.

When stimulation and sexual excitement build, the brain triggers muscles around the base of the penis to contract forcibly sending out sperm and other collected liquids in the form of semen during orgasm.

After an orgasm, the brain again sends a signal to the genitals telling the muscles to relax, releasing the blood and allowing the penis to become soft (or flaccid again).

There is no "normal" penis size or shape, just as there is no "normal" when it comes to vagina or anus size or shape. The bottom line is: for most people, satisfying sexual experiences have very little to do with the size or shape of the organs, and a lot more to do with what you do with it (and with whom).

# CHAPTER FIVE
# BODY IMAGE

**B**ody image involves the way we see ourselves in our minds and in our mirrors, and the way we think and feel about what we see.[1]

This is severely impacted by the cultures we live and grow up in. Technology, medical advances, and the media can also have enormous impact on an individual person's perception of their own body. Most people are more concerned with their appearance than they may care to admit, and whether that image is positive or negative, real or distorted, interferes with not only how we feel about ourselves, but also how we interact with the rest of the world.

Negative feelings about our bodies can cause anxiety, self-consciousness, and shame that can leave us feeling disconnected from ourselves. Positive feelings about our bodies can give us confidence, comfort, and a feeling of control.

What we feel and think when we look at ourselves in the mirror or a selfie can be impacted by our sex, gender, orientation, age, peers, relationship status, our level of activity, the media we consume, and bigger-picture, cultural issues such as race, religion, parents, and politics. Everyone experiences body dissatisfaction at some point in their lives, and if you identify as trans there may be times when the volume of those feelings can feel quite high.

For everyone—though especially those on the trans spectrum—it is important to understand that you are so much more than the body you were born into. Your body is part of who you are, but it does not define you.

**Gender dysphoria** is the medical diagnosis typically given to a person whose assigned birth gender is not the same as the one with which they identify.[2] Gender dysphoria used to be called gender identity disorder, though as the problem is not actually a mental disorder (it's about the confusion, pain, and distress caused by the disconnect between a person's physical body and their internal sense of themselves), it was changed.

According to the American Psychiatric Association's *Diagnostic and Statistical Manual of Mental Disorders* (DSM), the term refers to children, adolescents, and adults who experience a real and ongoing disconnect (or difference) between the sex assigned to them at birth and their internal sense of that gender.[3]

Gender dysphoria and body image issues are cousins in a way. For trans people, HRT (and/or surgeries) can help you feel more comfortable with your own body by more closely aligning your external physique to your internal sense of self, and lessen your sense of gender dysphoria. However, even after transition, there may still be bigger-picture, cultural standards of beauty or attractiveness and/or more personal expectations and desires about your outward appearance that you do not meet. These standards and expectations (as well as your desire and ability to meet them) can change over time, but it is important to remember that hormones/surgeries can change your body but not necessarily your body image. If you identify as trans, and find that you are struggling with body image problems after you begin to transition, counseling can help.

Red flags that signal issues around negative body image can include habitual negative self-talk, holding unrealistic standards of bodies or beauty, making poor choices in order to fit in or be accepted, excessive exercise, and disordered eating habits.

Disordered eating typically takes two forms. One form of **eating disorder** is binging and purging (referred to as bulimia) in which someone gorges on large amounts of food, then forces it back out of their body either by making themselves throw it up afterward or through the use of laxatives. The second form is starvation (also referred to as anorexia), causing a difficulty in gaining and maintaining weight due to fear and/or a disturbance in the way someone sees or feels about their body.

More than one million Americans have eating disorders; the vast majority of them identify as female.[4] In our society, women (cis and trans) are judged more often and more critically on their appearance than men. American standards of attractiveness are higher and less flexible for gay men than straight men as well, so don't be fooled into thinking that eating disorders do not have an impact on men (cis and trans) as well.

Statistically, 10 percent of eating-disordered people identify as male.[5] The "boy" versions of these issues are (only somewhat jokingly) referred to as "manorexia" or "boylimia," but they do exist and are very serious.[6]

Eating disorders can be extremely damaging to your body—in fact 10 percent of people with eating disorders die within ten years,[7] so it is important you speak to your doctor if you have concerns about your body, if you find yourself not eating for long periods of time, or if you regularly make yourself purge.

Negative body images are more prominent in anyone who was teased about their body as children, anyone who suffered from gender dysphoria, and both those who are overweight and those who are very athletic.

Developing a regular exercise habit and surrounding yourself with a diversity of other people by joining in teams, groups, or clubs can help reduce stress and anxiety about your body. Acknowledging the things you do well, striving to be excellent (rather than perfect) while you do them, and putting your energy into friends who do the same can help maintain a positive body image.

Remember that every body is different, including yours, and be proud of that.

If you are trans, some additional things you can do to create and maintain a positive body image include:

- Getting comfortable with your body. Altering your dress, presentation, and hairstyle is one way to do this (see chapter 12).

- Thinking of it as "my body" rather than "my male body" or "my female body."

- Learning to hold traditional ideas of femininity and masculinity lightly, and creating your own definitions out of them.

- Remembering that your body does not define you as a whole person.

- Appreciating what your body can do—your physical abilities and talents. There may be things you don't like about your body, but there are things that you can do with it that you can appreciate and be proud of.

- Learning about yourself, figuring things out about your life, and discovering who you are inside your skin, can pave the way to be happy about your outsides as well.

Feeling good about your body, regardless of your gender identity, isn't always easy. But by focusing on the things that make you powerful, unique, and special, you can find ways of appreciating and accepting yourself as well as your body. If you find yourself struggling to do this, consider finding a therapist to help.

# PART TWO
# "TRUE COLORS"

**Sex and gender are different things.**

Your sex is associated with your physical parts and biological status, assigned to you at birth, as male or female. It is a reproductive category, referring to physical attributes such as sex chromosomes, gonads (testicles and ovaries), hormones, internal reproductive structures, and genitalia—the "boy parts" and the "girl parts." Sex is where you are on the spectrum of male to female.

Your gender is where you are on the spectrum of masculine to feminine. It is a social phenomenon having to do with societal cultural expectations about how a person of a given sex "ought" to behave. The term "gender" is often used to refer to the ways that people act, interact, or feel about themselves—how "guy-like" or "chick-like" you are—and it has nothing to do with what kind of genitals you have. Instead, it has to do with the time period, family, culture, and geographical location in which you live. It can change depending on the situation, time, and place. Masculinity and femininity are cultural inventions.

## CHAPTER SIX
# IDENTITY AND THE SPECTRUM

**S**exual identity is your identity with respect to the plumbing with which you were born (or alter later through surgery)—the physical parts, including the hormones, the chromosomes, and other body characteristics associated with males and females.[1]

One of the identities on this spectrum would be intersex. An intersex person

- may have both male and female biological characteristics;

- may be chromosomally (internally) one sex, while physically (externally) another;

- may have biological sex characteristics that cannot be classified as either male or female.

The word *hermaphrodite* has been used to refer to people with both male and female sexual organs, but this term is misleading, stigmatizing, and should never be used. There are no actual human hermaphrodites. The preferred term for someone with atypical combinations of features that are usually considered male or female is intersex.

**Gender identity** refers to one's sense of oneself as a **man**, a **woman**, both, or neither. **Transgender** or **cisgender** can be descriptors of this phenomenon.[2]

Transgender (often abbreviated to "trans") is an umbrella term used to describe people whose gender identity (sense of themselves as male or female) or gender expression may differ from the body shape and parts they were born with. Examples of this include a girl born with "boy parts," or someone who feels like a boy on the inside, but was "born with a girl's body."

The opposite of this is cisgender (pronounced "sis-gender," and often abbreviated to "cis"). This is when your sense of yourself as a male or a female matches your body's biology.

An often-confused term with cisgender is **gender conforming**. This refers to a person whose gender expression is consistent with cultural norms for their gender—boys and men whose dress, demeanor, and deeds are "masculine," and girls and women whose dress, demeanor, and deeds are "feminine." It's confusing because not all cisgender people are gender conforming, and not all transgender people are gender nonconforming: for example, a trans man may have a very masculine gender expression, but so might a cisgender woman.

Other gender identities on the spectrum include **genderqueer** and **genderfluid** or **agender**; these are people who may think of themselves as

- being a third sex—between both male and female;

- being beyond or falling completely outside the gender binary;

- moving back and forth between genders;

- genderless—neither male nor female, and/or rejecting the idea of a gender binary altogether.

**Your gender identity is connected to,
but not dependent on, your sexual identity.**

**Transsexual** is an older, mostly out of date term to describe transgender people who have engaged in hormone therapies and/or surgical procedures (called gender reassignment or gender confirmation surgeries) to live as members of the gender opposite to the sex they were born. While some people still use it as an identity label, most people who were assigned one sex at birth, but identify with another, generally prefer the term transgender (or simply, trans) to describe themselves. Because not everyone does, can, or wants to use some kind of medical intervention to change their chemistry or physical structure, the term transsexual is considered more of a medical term, rather than a social one, and is typically only used by people outside of the trans community. You may also see the alternative spelling, "transexual" (with one S). Some people use this rarer (and technically, incorrect) spelling as a way to de-medicalize the term.

Transition is the process of making changes to your appearance or biology in order to live as a member of the gender opposite to the sex you were born (see chapter 12).

People assigned male at birth who wish to live and be recognized as women can also refer to themselves as male-to-female (**MTF**) transsexuals, or trans women. People assigned female at birth who wish to live and be recognized as men can also refer to themselves as female-to-male (**FTM**) transsexuals, or trans men. (*Note*: it's trans man, not "transman"— like they're a superhero or something.)

Other transgender people may simply prefer to be referred to as a man or a woman, without any qualifiers or modifiers.

The estimated population of transgender people in the United States is now 1.4 million adults according to The Williams Institute, a division of the UCLA School of Law, and the United States' leading researcher on LGBT demographics. According to a 2016 report, transgender people now comprise 0.6 percent of the country's total population.[3] That is slightly more than the percentage of the American population that has been on active military duty at any given time (0.5 percent).[4] To be clearer, there are more transgender people in America than there are people actively serving in the US military.

Gender identity and sexual identity are different: transgender people can be gay, straight, or bisexual; masculine, feminine, or androgynous. You can't tell if someone is trans just by their appearance. It's important to remember that not everyone whose appearance or behavior is gender atypical or gender nonconforming identifies as transgender.

---

## LGBTW . . . Vocabulary

We are now evolving to a new understanding that there is no true gender binary—viewing gender as either male or female, with no integration, middle-ground, or "third-space" options. The concept of a gender binary is considered to be problematic and limiting for those who do not fit neatly and conveniently into those two, simplistic, either-or categories.

In reality, there are more than just two distinct genders, with many shades of gray in between "male" and "female." The concept of gender as a simple and limited thing with only two parts is inaccurate and oppressive, because it does not take into account the diversity of gender identity and variance in gender expression in people.

A new vocabulary is emerging to solve challenges around fluid, mixed, and separate identities. It is socially acceptable (in fact, encouraged) for people to ask, "What pronouns do you prefer?"

There are many options in terms of answers that can go beyond the expected "he/him/his," or "she/her/hers," including:

- "they/them/theirs,"
- "ey/em/eirs,"
- "ze/hir/hirs," or
- "ze/zir/zirs."

As in:

"They are going to the movies. I am going with them. We are taking their car."

"Ey is going to the movies. I am going with em. We are taking eir car." or

"Ze is going to the movies. I am going with zir. We are taking zir car."

Alternative pronouns are becoming increasingly hyper-individuated, and the Internet has helped to create loads of variations on this dynamic, important (and sometimes confusing) concept.

In all of the above cases, pronouns should not be based on the shape of one's genitals, the clothes one wears, or any other outside detail, but instead on what one prefers to be called.

Because culture and the medical professions have changed so much, there is also some vocabulary that is now on The No-No List:

**The No-No List:**

- "Post-Op" (for someone who has had gender reassignment surgery).
- "Pre-Op" (for someone who has not).

Medical intervention is only one part of transition, and the procedures are not chosen or affordable by all transgender people, so emphasizing the presence (or not) of surgical operations can be alienating and considered rude.

- "Sex change"

The operations are referred to as gender confirmation surgery (GCS) or gender reassignment surgery (GRS) (see chapter 12).

- "Transgendered"

Most people are shying away from the "ed" on the end of the word, mostly because it carries an implication that something has happened to a trans person to make them trans, as opposed to a legitimate identity that the person was born with. It could be argued that people can be referred to as *transgendered* (just as one is simply *gendered* at birth), but many individuals may have semantic issues, it can be considered quite offensive in the trans community, and GLAAD recently made a statement[5] in clear favor of leaving off the "ed" both grammatically and philosophically.

- "Tranny"
- "SheMale"
- "HeShe"
- "It"

These words are pornified and vulgar and have no place in civilized conversation. They are used by ignorant and bigoted people to target transgender people either to delegitimize their experiences or to dehumanize them as people. Though it is true that some transgender people have taken back the word *tranny* (as gay culture has with "fag" and lesbians have with "dyke"), it is *only* appropriate if you are transgender yourself (and even then, many find it offensive).

## LGBTW . . . The Singular "They"

The Singular "They" involves using the (historically multiple) pronoun "they" as a gender-neutral pronoun to refer to a single person, instead of "he" or "she." As both our language and conceptualization of sexuality and gender evolve, it has become clear that the binary references of "he" and "she" don't fit, represent, or include everyone anymore.

The American Dialect Society appointed the singular, gender-neutral pronoun, "they" as 2015's Word of the Year; however, The Singular "They" has been used for a long time for either a person who does not fit cleanly into the binary of male or female or in situations in which a person's gender is unclear or unknown—even Shakespeare and Jane Austen used "they" to refer to only one person.

Though possibly confusing to some, and potentially annoying to others, these drawbacks are far outweighed by the benefits of The Singular "They," including more inclusive reference, general respect, and avoiding sexist and inaccurate misgendering mishaps.

Misgendering isn't seen as a typo anymore—it's seen as a refusal to offer another person basic, ground-level dignity. Once you know someone's preference, it is polite to do your best to respect that person's choices.

That being said, many good people struggle, and (as maddening as it can be) some people are going to need time and reminders before they catch on and catch up.

With a bit of conscious effort and only slightly more practice, The Singular "They" can become a regular and seamless part of your everyday communication, if it isn't already.

Now back to our regularly scheduled chapter on the gender spectrum.

**Transvestites**, or **cross-dressers**, wear clothing typical of the opposite sex to varying degrees. Some cross-dress to express cross-gender feelings, some do it for fun, some for emotional comfort or sexual arousal. The majority of cross-dressers are straight males. Transvestites may or may not also identify as transgender.

**Drag queens** (males) and **drag kings** (females) live part-time as members of the other sex, primarily as performers. The majority of drag performers identify as gay or lesbian, and may or may not identify as transgender.

**Identity and expression (or orientation) are also different things.**

# EXPRESSION AND THE SPECTRUM

S exual expression or sexual orientation refer to which sex you choose to be sexual with, and its relationship to your own. It refers to one's sexual attraction to men, women, both, or neither: where you are on the spectrum of **gay** to **straight**. **Bisexuality** is an orientation somewhere in the middle of that spectrum.[1]

**Heterosexuality** is physical and/or emotional attraction to people of the opposite sex: when a man and a woman have a romantic or sexual relationship. Heterosexuality is also called "being straight." This is a strange term that implies that not only is heterosexuality the norm for most people (which is true), but also that anyone who is not heterosexual is "bent" (which is *not* true).

In most societies, heterosexuality is the most obvious, accepted, and visually dominant behavior with regard to sex. It is the primary way that our species reproduces, the most default sexual orientation, and the one you are most likely to see depicted in television and film.

**Homosexuality** is the romantic or sexual attraction to someone of the same sex. Though the word *gay* is used in general to describe this, gay typically refers to a male who is attracted to another male, and "lesbian" is the preferred term for a female who is attracted to another female.

Same-sex sex is a phenomenon that has been observed in hundreds of species[2]; mammals and sea life, including lions, dolphins, and killer whales, even birds and worms. In fact, no species has been found in which homosexual behavior does not exist (with the exception of species that never have sex at all or that are hermaphroditic).

The term GLBTQ stands for gay, lesbian, bisexual, transgender, and queer (generally meaning "not straight" but could also include aspects of gender fluidity) or questioning (meaning "I haven't made up my mind yet," and again, can refer to sex and/or gender). LGBTQ is another version of this initialism, and the two terms are often used interchangeably depending on personal or political preference (they are used interchangeably throughout this book).

The number of letters and symbols can be impractical or confusing, and the order can be arbitrary and *very* personal for some people—because identity is loaded and important and even individual communities are not always united. You may also see an A (for Asexuals and/or Allies), I for Intersex, O for Other, or 2S for the First Nation/Native American concept of Two-Spirit. Sometimes even symbols such as * or + are used in an effort to include a multitude of other specific groups, cohorts, and minorities. It can look sometimes like your autocorrect may have had a stroke, but the whole point of the initialism is inclusion and identification, so pick your favorite, aim for respect, and don't be afraid to ask when you encounter a term or string of letters you're not familiar with.

Approximately 3.5 percent of the US population identifies in the GLBT range.[3] That works out to approximately nine million people; however, this number may be misleading. The figure most likely includes only people who are comfortable with their homosexuality (and are "out"), since people who are not out don't tend to publicly identify. "Out" means that you are open about your sexuality and tell people you are G, L, B, T, or Q.

**Bisexuality** refers to attraction to both genders, being sexually attracted to both men and women.

In 1948, sexologist Alfred Kinsey created the Kinsey scale,[4] a questionnaire that served to rate a person's attraction and behavior with regard to sex along a continuum. The questionnaire asked people to rate on a scale of 0–6 whom they're attracted to physically, whom they're attracted to emotionally, and what they've done about it.

Kinsey found that most people have both heterosexual and homosexual thoughts and feelings, and that the majority of people engage in sex with people of both sexes at some point in their lives. This suggested that most people are some flavor of bisexual.

Most contemporary research agrees with this, and describes sexual identity as being very fluid—a continuum scale, rather than closed categories. This idea meshes with the general understanding that sexuality develops and can change in many ways over a person's lifetime. Most people do not stay in the exact same place on the scale for their entire life. Very few people think, feel, or do the same things sexually when they are fifteen as they do when they are twenty, forty, or sixty.

Most sex educators tend to reach the same general conclusions as Kinsey: heterosexuality, bisexuality, and homosexuality make up a sexual identity continuum. Although they might gravitate to either the "gay" or "straight" end of this continuum, most people float somewhere in the middle, and many, many men and women experiment with same-sex sex at some point.

**Asexuality**, also known as "ace," is generally associated with a lack of sexual interest or desire.

Like being straight or gay, asexuality is considered a sexual orientation. Different than homosexuality or heterosexuality, asexuality is not about what one does, it's about what one does not do. Approximately 1 percent of the world's population identifies as asexual.[5]

Being abstinent is different than being asexual. Abstinence is not engaging in sexual activity at all. It is a conscious choice made for personal, philosophical, situational, cultural, or spiritual reasons.

Though asexual people are often abstinent from sexual activity, asexuality is a lack of sexual attraction, not the same as ignoring or repressing one's sexual desires. It's the difference between being on a cleanse, a fast, or a diet and not being hungry.

All humans are unique and individual, and sexual orientations (including asexuality) exist on spectrums.

Some people with low or lower sexual drive also identify as part of the ace community, and many asexual people still identify as lesbian, gay, straight, or bi. **Gray-asexual** means that a person experiences sexual attraction, but not very often or only a bit when they do. **Demisexual** describes a person who only feels sexual attraction to people with whom a close emotional bond has been formed.

People can completely separate romantic attraction from physical attraction as well, with **heteroromantic**, being romantic (but not physical) attraction to people of the opposite sex, and **homoromantic**, being romantic (but not physical) attraction to people of the same sex.

None of these things conflict with asexuality in any way. There are loads of ways an asexual person might be in relationships with others without sexual attraction being part of it, including dating and falling in love.

This means that someone who identifies as asexual can be:

- Abstinent completely.

- Sexually active with themselves through masturbation.

- Affectionate, including kissing and cuddling.

- Identify as gay, straight, or bi.

- Sexually active with partners for reasons like pleasing a partner or wanting to have children.

- Committed to a partner, in long-term relationships, even married.

## The Other No-No List

- "A Gay"

is considered depersonalizing. They are not "a gay." They are gay. Like they are smart. Or they are funny. Or they are tired of having their individuality denied by annoying terms like, "a gay."

- "Fag"
- "Dyke"
- "Queen"
- "Lez"
- "Homo"

These terms should be used only if you are "in the club" (or at least close enough to be invited to the bake sale). And, even then, you should tread carefully so as not to appear insensitive.

- "Homosexual"

Gay and lesbian are the preferred terms, as homosexual sounds too "medical," has been used to pathologize queer people in the past, and places an unnecessary emphasis on the sex part (instead of the person part).

- "Queer"

Though this and other terms have been reclaimed by parts of the gay community, they are still off limits to certain people and situations. It can be acceptable as long as it's said in a nice way, and generally as an adjective not as a noun. Again, club membership is recommended.

- "Lifestyle"

An inaccurate and increasingly outdated term that implies that the lives of gay people are (1) all the same, and (2) totally different than their straight counterparts. Though there *is* a culture, with its own art and literature, and a community of gay-identified and friendly businesses, holidays, and politics, there is no "lifestyle," just as there is no true *straight* lifestyle. People don't go straight grocery shopping, they go grocery shopping. People don't get gay married, they just get married.

- "That's so gay."

It's more popular (and delivers less blunt trauma) than the classics "faggot" or "lesbo," though it's no less hateful or harmful. Often used to describe things stupid, weird, not-good-enough, or otherwise unsavory, it's a gateway drug to more serious offenses—normalizing "gay" as something inherently wrong or distasteful.

**Gender expression** refers to one's dress, demeanor, and deeds, the relationship of those things to one's sexual and gender identity, and how they are interpreted by others. **Masculine** and **feminine** are typical adjectives related to gender expression. **Androgynous** is an example of an identity within the spectrum of gender expression.[6]

An androgynous person

- does not fit cleanly into typical masculine and feminine roles, and/or

- is able to draw from both traditionally masculine and feminine qualities.

- combines masculine and feminine qualities in non-traditional ways.

Many people are gender nonconforming and express their gender in ways that are not typical or conventional in terms of what we have decided things like "masculine" mean or what "feminine" looks like

**Your gender expression is connected to, but not dependent on, your sexual orientation.**

People generally experience sex, gender, orientation, and expression as different things. While aspects of biological sex are the same across different cultures, aspects of sexuality, such as gender and expression, may not be.

Self-identity and sexual orientation both form slowly over time and in the context of life experiences. Sexuality is very fluid, meaning how a person identifies today is not necessarily how they did in the past or will in the future.

No one should feel pressured to label themselves until they are ready, but it is important to find someone to talk to about any troubling thoughts and feelings. Talking to a trusted friend, adult, doctor, or teacher is especially important if you have felt targeted, threatened, harmed, or abused because of your identity or orientation.

# PART THREE
# "I'M COMING OUT"

There are many theories about how sexuality develops, but one thing is for certain: sexuality is no more a choice than ear shape, musical ability, or height.

Don't believe me? Ask the American Psychiatric Association, American Academy of Pediatrics, American Counseling Association, American Association of School Administrators, American Federation of Teachers, American School Health Association, Interfaith Alliance, National Association of School Psychologists, National Association of Social Workers, National Education Association, and the World Health Organization.[1]

Like ear shape, musical ability, and height, sexuality is most likely a combination of biology and environment.[2] Biological influences on whether someone is straight, gay, both, neither, or somewhere in between include genes, prenatal hormones, and the structure of the brain. The environmental pieces can be more obvious in some ways and harder to pin down in others. Social and cultural stigmas, religion, politics, media, and laws get in the way of people being able to deal honestly with their own (and others') sexuality.

# CHAPTER EIGHT
# COMING OUT

"**C**oming out" is the process of accepting and being open about one's sexual orientation, particularly when one's orientation is not straight. This is part of being healthy, being true to yourself, and being the most "you" you can be.[1]

The first stage of coming out is coming out to one's self—exploring and deciding where you are in that huge gray area between straight and gay, then acknowledging your own sexual orientation.

The opposite of being out is called "closeted." When one is gay, staying in the closet means choosing not to disclose parts of your identity to others, and is not the healthiest of choices (understandable and necessary at times for safety or financial reasons—but ultimately, not the healthiest).

Coming out can seem unfair in the sense that straight people do not have to sit down with friends and loved ones to explain to them that they like the opposite sex and then answer those people's questions. Although it is not unusual or unhealthy to keep aspects of our personal and sexual lives private, fighting against who you are, pretending to be someone you are not, or living a life in which you have to keep secrets or tell lies is exhausting, and cannot be done for long periods of time without causing problems. And remember, just because coming out can be necessary or helpful, that does not mean that people who are not straight need to tell anyone specific or gory details about their sex lives or practices.

For not-straight/not-cis people, coming out gives you the space to act and speak openly about your life, relationships, and activities without having to self-consciously screen your personal information and the audience you are sharing it with. Coming out also helps queer people avoid being autopiloted into other people's assumptions about what you do, who you date, and how you identify.

**The rules of coming out are very similar to that of a swimming pool.**[2]

**First of all, have fun.** Be proud and enjoy yourself, celebrate who you are, and surround yourself with people who want to do the same.

**Wear sunscreen.** Well, OK, not sunscreen, but do protect yourself. Safer not-straight sex can be different than what you have been taught, seen, tried, or even had to think about. Ask questions and educate yourself before you jump in and start swimming.

**Wade into the pool.** Opening up to one or two trusted friends or family members can help to slowly gather support as you build your confidence and is often a better way to start the coming out process than just jumping right in.

**No running.** Go slowly. Be prepared for some people to be shocked and possibly upset—particularly parents—and be gentle with them. Most parents experience a range of reactions when a child comes out. These reactions can range from "Does this mean I will never have grandchildren?" to worrying about your safety, to their own biases and prejudices from growing up in a different generation or culture. It is difficult (though important) to try not to take these reactions too personally.

**Be patient.** Give each person you come out to a few days to digest the new information, and invite them to ask questions (because they might not know how to, or may be afraid of upsetting or offending you). Don't be too patient, though. After a few weeks, if your friends are still being weird about it, move on. Author and podcast host Dan Savage advocates that parents should get a year to freak out, be sad, to wrap their brains around stuff, to slip up and say stupid things, to ask uncomfortable or even inappropriate questions. One year. Then they need to get up, get over it, get on board.

Moving forward in your own life in an authentic way is the highest priority. That being said, there may be family members, friends, or other people in your life who may need longer, and you may be put in a position in which you may need to decide if waiting for them to accept you is important enough to you and possible without compromising your own growth.

**Keep an eye out for others.** Do not be surprised to hear a few "Me, toos" (a few "Polos" to your "Marco"), when you start coming out. It's hard to know who else is in the pool until you get your head underwater.

**Safety first.** Take care of yourself and surround yourself with resources and information, such as the It Gets Better Project (itgetsbetter.org) or your school's Gay-Straight Alliance (GSA)—sometimes also known as a QSA (Queer Straight Alliance).

**Don't splash** those who are not in the pool. It is never cool to out someone else.

Coming out helps build self-esteem and a capacity for intimacy. But it can be very stressful, sometimes harming self-esteem in the process. Dealing with gay thoughts and feelings (let alone coming out) is a difficult process, and can result in feelings of isolation and societal stigmas stemming from fear, bigotry, and hatred.

Thirty percent of gays and lesbians report that they have attempted suicide at some point in their life.[3] Most gay people prior to the 1970s were closeted because of fear of being mistreated or victimized; being gay was even considered a mental illness until the mid-1970s.[4]

Today, it is much safer for someone to come out and be out, although many gay people still have to struggle with negative stereotypes, media misinformation, and fear—all of which is called "homophobia."

---

### LGBTW . . . Homophobia

Homophobia is fear and apprehension of gay people, experience, or things. Hatred of gay people can come from that fear. That fear comes from ignorance, and/or from people's reactions to their own gay thoughts and feelings.

Homophobia is a social disease, like racism, sexism, or other kinds of bigotry. It is unfair, harmful, and too often becomes violent. This kind of violence is called "gay bashing," and is considered a hate crime.[5] It's the same as when someone is victimized because of the color of their skin, gender identity, or their religious beliefs.

---

There are some terms that are considered homophobic: "fag" (or "faggot"), "dyke," and "queer." Like "nigger" and other racist slurs, these words are designed to insult and humiliate people based on qualities they cannot control or change. It is never cool to shame, tease, be hateful to, or treat someone differently for something they have no control over.

Also, as with "nigger" and other racist slurs, some minority groups have attempted to reclaim the negative terms, using them amongst and in reference to themselves as a way to lessen the impact and pain those words are associated with. It is only acceptable to use those taken-back terms if you are "in the club," like black guys calling one another "nigga," or gay girls calling each other "dyke." If you are not in a particular club (or close enough to someone who is invited to the picnic), using these terms is extremely insensitive and disrespectful, and should be avoided.

Like "retarded," using "gay" as an insult (as in: "That shirt is so gay") should be considered a very big no-no. People who use these offensive terms as insults should probably be avoided, as well.

Although the vast majority of educated therapists and researchers state that sexual orientation is unchangeable, there are still people who believe the opposite—that conversion (also called reparative therapy) is possible and effective. These people believe that people can choose their sexuality (people can't). Some try to use prayer, counseling, and even drugs to try to "cure" gay people. These techniques are never aimed at straight people.

Therapy can be helpful for people who are troubled by their sexuality, or are struggling emotionally or socially, but according to the American Psychiatric Association, there is no evidence that any treatment can change a homosexual person's feelings for others of the same sex. There is no published science-based evidence supporting the efficacy of reparative therapy as a treatment to change anyone's sexual orientation.[6]

Changing a person's sexual orientation would not simply be about changing behavior. It would involve altering someone's emotional, romantic, and sexual feelings, as well as re-creating one's entire self-concept and social identity. People can change their behavior, but not their internal experience.

# COMING OUT BI

S tudies show that 1.8 percent of the population identifies as bi—that's
more than gay and lesbian combined, at 1.7 percent.[1] Ironically, the
same study reported that bisexuals are less than half as likely to be
out as gays and lesbians.

Coming out as bisexual is different than coming out as gay in many
ways.

A binary is assumed in relationships, and there is a cultural assumption that if you're dating someone of the opposite sex, you're straight.
And if you're dating someone of the same sex, you're gay. No one ever
assumes that someone is bisexual. So unless your sexual identity just happens to come up organically in casual conversation, bisexuals are often
left in a position in which they must choose to (1) either actively correct
someone's assumption or (2) just go with someone's assumptions. Both
can be exhausting.

Some people just have a hard time understanding bisexuality for some
reason. People understand if you enjoy both steak and fish. It's not considered weird if you happen to enjoy both cake and pie. Liking cats and dogs
is OK as well as enjoying both Instagram and Twitter. Even both Taylor
and Kanye on the same playlist won't necessarily raise an eyebrow . . . but
if you say you like to kiss girls *and* boys, some people may react as if the
gravity was just turned off.

Then there's this thing called bi erasure. Bi erasure is a phenomenon
in which bisexuality is explained away, distrusted, or treated as if it doesn't
exist. Unlike leprechauns or the Easter Bunny, bisexuality *is* an actual
thing. However, many bisexuals face judgment and alienation from both
sides of the fence they sometimes straddle.

There is a stereotype in gay culture that bisexuals will eventually default to an opposite sex partner because it's easier/safer. On the straight side of the fence, bi is sometimes just rounded up to gay—as if "bisexuals" are only half out of the closet and will eventually come out as gay. This is perpetuated primarily by popular/straight culture's unspoken rule that bi-girls are hot (but will always end up with the boy), and that bi-boys are always "secret-gay."

It is also perpetuated by gay culture's belief that bisexuals have an easier go of things because they do not necessarily have to be out in as obvious a way as someone who identifies as lesbian or gay.

Unfortunately, bi privilege is real—especially for bisexuals who primarily date, engage in long-term relationships with, or marry people of the opposite sex. A bisexual who is not obvious or out does not face the same risks of rejection, oppression, and violence that an out or obvious gay man or lesbian may face. Though some people do come out as bisexual, then identify as something else later as their relationship to their sexuality evolves, and some bisexuals may go through their day-to-day existence being assumed-straight (thereby experiencing more positive and/or fewer negative interactions than their gay peers), the concept of bi privilege is still wrongly used as a weapon against bisexuals within the LGBT community. Coming out proudly as bisexual (if that is how you identify) helps to reduce bi ignorance and change some of these stereotypes.

## CHAPTER TEN
# COMING OUT ACE

Many of the people in your life may not be aware of asexuality as a valid sexual orientation. This may be due to ignorance, not necessarily anti-asexual bias—the concept can be very difficult for some people to wrap their brains around.

It can be frustrating to be the first person of any identity that's open about it in a social group, and being the spokesperson for asexuality might not be your idea of fun, but the people you are close to may appreciate having a better understanding of asexuality and what that means in someone's actual life.

Coming out as asexual can

- allow people to be more open and honest about their lives and interests.

- keep others from making incorrect assumptions about them that might be uncomfortable or awkward to deal with.

- help people feel closer to friends and family, knowing that they've shared a core component of their identity with someone else.

- be rewarding to be the first person of a certain identity that's open about it in a social group.

That being said, you aren't ever required to come out to everyone in your life, or to explain why you aren't in or looking for a relationship to the people that you do.

If you don't want to get into explaining asexuality for those who don't know the term (or don't feel like justifying your choices to people who ask), it's OK to answer awkward questions with vagueness or a deflection. Responding to questions with something like, "I'm focusing on [work, school, hobbies]," or "Sex/romance isn't a priority in my life . . . " can get the idea across without relying on any specific terminology.

There may be the exuberant bestie, the parent-who-wants-to-be-a-grandparent, or that over-involved coworker/roommate/bestie-in-law who desperately wants to set you up on a date. In that situation, you may need to say something more assertive like, "It sounds like having a partner/relationship works for you/is your thing, but that is not true for me, and I'd appreciate it if you would stop trying to change my mind." (It would be extremely rude for any reasonable person to keep pushing after that level of clarity!)

If you do identify as ace and find yourself in a non-sexual, romantic relationship (or a relationship with a low level of physical contact)—especially with a person who does not identify as ace, it is very important to be clear about what your goals and expectations are from the relationship. As many relationships start out G or PG, most graduate to PG-13 or R in terms of sexual contact over time. If that is not your goal, it is important to communicate that in case that *is* the other person's (understandable) expectation for the future.

Gaining consent in terms of *not* having sexual contact is just as respectful and important as gaining consent in order to have sexual contact.

Online asexual communities and resources like Asexuality.org can be a big help; there are plenty of people who are willing to share their knowledge experiences in the ace community.

# COMING OUT TRANS

Coming out as gay, lesbian, or bi is the process of accepting and being open about one's sexual orientation. This is part of being healthy, being true to yourself, and being the most "you" that you can be. For trans people, being healthy, being true to themselves, and being the most "they" that they can be means living as or transitioning to their authentic gender. This may or may not include having others know you are trans.[1]

Coming out is about being healthy and true to yourself. Coming out as gay is about telling. Coming out as trans is often more about showing. This is often done through dress and modifying one's appearance. Trans people can also seek medical interventions, such as hormones and surgery, to make their bodies as congruent as possible with their gender. The process of changing from one gender to another is called transitioning (see chapter 12).

People who are attracted to women prior to transition generally continue to be attracted to women after transition, and people who are attracted to men prior to transition generally continue to be attracted to men after transition. That means, for example, that a person assigned male at birth who is attracted to females will still be attracted to females after making their transition, and may identify as lesbian (though the sexuality of a trans person can be as fluid as anyone else's).

It is important to understand that hormones and medical interventions do not make someone "more of a" man or change them into a "real" woman—they can only help someone feel more comfortable in their own skin.

Some people find hormones or medical procedures an important part of their comfort level with their bodies, *and* there are many trans people who feel and find themselves completely comfortable with their gender expression without any HRT or surgery at all.

The interventions that are available change rapidly as the science and culture evolve. If/when you find yourself considering *any* sort of medical intervention, this writer suggests

- Doing diligent research.

- Talking to your doctor about your findings.

- Forming a realistic plan that works for you.

- Participating in talk therapy with someone both knowledgeable and comfortable with the subject of gender.

- Surrounding yourself with supportive people.

Coming and being "out" is a process that is continual. Although not being out for extended periods of time can cause problems, it is important to remember to keep context in mind. For people who live in a place, culture, or family in which an alternative sexuality or identity is unwelcome, it may be smarter or safer to wait to come out until circumstances change. As an adult, you will have more opportunity and ability to create your safe spaces than you do as an adolescent.

Sometimes, when people think about coming out, they imagine only two states: being closeted or being 100 percent out to 100 percent of everyone. This is not true. Many people who want to disclose the truth of their sexual orientation or gender identity will choose to come out to a few close friends or family members first, before possibly expanding that to acquaintances, schoolmates, coworkers, and community members, or by being visibly active in a way that might do the outing for them.

There's a huge difference, though, in deliberately telling everyone you know and mentioning it to a couple of people you're close to, as it comes up organically in conversation. Even if you don't want to come out publicly to everyone in your life, you may find it helpful to do so to a few close friends.

For any given identity, some people really feel it as a core part of themselves, and want to be visible members of that community. Others are happy having a label for their own personal self-understanding with no outside acknowledgment. Your process is yours, and it is important and healthy to move forward, but in the beginning it is OK to move slowly and important to stay safe.

## LGBTW . . . Coming Out to Parents

Whether gay, lesbian, bi, or trans, if you are old enough to be reading this book, and have not come out to your parents, there is a decent chance they already know, wonder, or suspect.

- They might think that if you don't talk about it, none of you will have to deal with it.

- They might hope you grow out of it or it's some kind of phase.

- They might do this for selfish or biased reasons.

- More likely it is done out of ignorance or a legitimate attempt to spare you the difficult task of coming out/transitioning.

At some point most people do come out to their family. Coming out to family means adjustment—changes in the family relationships. Every family has different beliefs, values, and feelings. Beliefs, values, and feelings can all change with time and experience.

It's important to keep in mind that your folks may hold the notion that if you are queer, that they somehow "failed" as your parent. You must let them know that they didn't . . . and that you still love them.

**Other tips for coming out to your family:**

- Avoid coming out to the family late in the evening, on a work or school night, when something obviously big is happening in their work or personal life, and during big events like holidays or family gatherings.

- There is no shame in prepping in advance: letting your parents know there is something big you'd like to discuss and "making an appointment" can help.

- Writing it out can be a good thing. Not sending an email or text, but a speech or letter (that you don't send, but can hold in your hand while you tell them) can help you get clear about what you want to say, and keep them from interrupting you until you are done.

- You can give your parents some resources for parental support like PFLAG or books—*Always My Child* by Kevin Jennings or *Oddly Normal* by John Schwartz are excellent and recommended choices.

- Don't let your parents find out through social media or some other third party. That can be a clear message that says, "I don't trust you," or "You are not important to me." Don't miss the chance to give your parents the opportunity to know you and be supportive. Some parents will fail at this, but most will not. It's important (unless you have clear evidence to the contrary) to give them the chance to do it right.

It's also important to remember that, if you think or feel that you will not be safe in your home if you are open and honest about your orientation, or identity, it may be safer or smarter to wait.

If anyone in your family becomes abusive in *any* way, for *any* reason—confide in an adult in a position of official authority like a teacher, school counselor, or your doctor.

## LGBTW . . . Coming Out at School

Your school should have zero tolerance for bullying and harassment of queer students, but enlisting your parents or other adult advocates to help you come out at school is a good idea. Identifying supportive adults at your school is important. Classrooms and doors with yellow and blue Human Rights Campaign (HRC) equality stickers, Safe Zone decals, or LGBT positive posters are signals that the occupants are supportive.

Other supportive people can be found in your school's gay-straight alliance. If your school has a gay-straight alliance, join. If they don't have one, think about creating one.

The GSA network lays out ten steps for starting a GSA/QSA at your school at gsanetwork.org.[2]

These include:

- Follow the guidelines at your school to establish a GSA/QSA the same way you would establish any other group or club.

- Find a teacher or staff member to serve as the faculty advisor.

- Tell the school administrators that you want to start a GSA/QSA chapter. (If an administrator is resistant to the GSA/QSA, let them know that forming a GSA/QSA club is protected under the Federal Equal Access Act.)

- Inform the school counselors about the group—they may know students who would be interested in joining.

- Pick a meeting place that offers some level of privacy or confidentiality.

- Let people know when and where, using bulletins, announcements, flyers, and word-of-mouth.

Gsanetwork.org has ideas and resources on how to start meetings as well as activities and goals once the group is started.

# TRANSITION

Transition has three primary components: social, medical, and legal.

Social transition is the part in which you start to culturally indicate your gender identity and make others aware of it. This can include:

- Changing your gender expression; your dress, demeanor, and deeds, including clothing and hairstyles, gait, and voice.

- Being/coming out to others about your gender identity and/or your transgender status.

- Telling others your preferred name, pronouns, and other gendered language preferences (like titles).

Medical transition is the part involving physical procedures to alter and match your physical body to your internal experience. This can include:

- Puberty blockage to delay puberty.

- Hormone Replacement Therapy (HRT), to help either feminize or masculinize your body.

- Gender Confirmation Surgery, which can include what is referred to as "top surgery" (breast augmentation or removal) or "bottom surgery" (altering genitalia).

**Legal transition** revolves around changing your identifying documents to accurately reflect your gender identity. This can include:

- Updating the name and gender category on your school and State IDs, state-issued driver's license, birth certificate, Social Security cards, and passports, as well as other identifying documents such as debit and library cards.

## Social Transition

If you are trans (and haven't already), at some point you are going to want to socially transition. It's often the first step to becoming your authentic self.

Unlike legal and medical transition, social transition can start as a solo activity or with a close group of trusted others, and is not necessarily dependent on other people, professionals, or paperwork. It also typically happens before the other two pieces of transition, which can make it both more exciting and more stressful.

It is definitely not necessary to socially transition all at once. Move at your own pace. Some people start alone or only in their own home, some try small, structured outings with a supportive friend or family member and slowly expand their circle of social transition, and some rip off the Band-Aid and go all-in.

It can be slightly easier for trans men to begin social transition than trans women, because in most western societies, it is generally considered OK for a "girl" to dress "like a boy," wearing shirts, jeans, baseball hats, and so forth. If you were assigned male at birth, it can be a bit more difficult, for example, to dress "like a girl," with barrettes or wearing skirts or makeup.

Adolescents—straight, trans, cis, and queer—try on different facets of identity as they figure out who they are. Social transition, in many ways, is simply an extension of that.

Back to my swimming metaphor for coming out (see chapter 8).

Before you get in the water and start splashing around, first figure out exactly what you feel comfortable doing: sitting on the edge and dipping your feet in? Sticking your head under, blowing some bubbles, then coming right back out? Or just doing a few laps?

Then, consider how you want to do it? Wading in slowly? Doggie paddling with some supportive floaties? A cannonball?

Some ideas (ranging from the shallower end of the pool to deeper waters) you could start with:

- Using "girls'" shampoo.

- Growing your hair out.

- Wearing nail polish.

- Wearing jewelry.

- Shaping your eyebrows.

- Wearing a skirt or dress.

- Using "men's" deodorant.

- Wearing "men's" shoes.

- Cutting your hair.

- Wearing masculine watches or ties.

- Changing your walk.

- Binding your breasts.

Many people choose to start social transition during the summer months. This can give you time away from the audience at school, a way to get some space or "go offline" without a lot of questions asked and no homework to worry about while you concentrate on yourself!

Some people also choose to change schools during social transition, claiming a clean slate and a fresh start, and a summertime transition means you get to enter a new school at the same time as a bunch of other people. This can help avoid some of the spotlight of being the new kid that enters midyear.

That being said—anyone (cis or trans, transitioned or not) entering a new school is going to be in a spotlight. People will notice you, be curious, and ask questions.

Keep it simple. Keep it truthful. Keep in mind that the whole point of transition is to be more you, so don't invent elaborate backstories that you will likely have to remember, back up, or untell.

Regardless of whether you remain at your school or move to a new one, people may or may not read you as trans. Rumors may go around, and if they do, your best reaction is not to react.

There is a high likelihood that the attention may move off of you quickly and onto the next interesting thing.

There is no shame in being trans.

There is no one who makes it through transition without dealing with ignorant, judgy, transphobic creeps. These are opportunities to build both character and muscle.

If someone confronts you in public about such rumors, your best defense is to

- Keep calm and maintain composure. (This can be particularly difficult if you are taking testosterone, but regardless, deep breathing helps.) If they are the only ones being inappropriate or making a scene, you can walk away being the bigger person (plus you will come off much better in the inevitable YouTube video).

- Remember your basic human rights—including your right to your own boundaries, to be treated with respect, to express yourself, to feel safe in the world, to protect yourself from harm and injustice.

- Do not engage unless you have to.

- If you do engage, do so without defensiveness. Responses can range from assertive to aggressive, for example, explaining your right to be there or flipping their inappropriate questions back at them ("What do *your* genitals look like?" / "When did *you* know you were a boy?").

- Keep your distance physically.

- Walk away when you can.

- Talk to someone with authority—whether it's at school or in a restaurant—to reinforce that such behavior is not OK, and there should be zero tolerance.

When socially transitioning at school, it is good practice to organize a meeting with school officials, the school's counselor, and your parents. Your regular doctor or therapist, team coaches, and supportive friends could also be invited.

Discuss with your school your chosen name (if it's changed) and your preferred pronouns. Then discuss how and when your school ID (and eventually your records) will be changed. You may need to sort out accommodations for P.E. classes and sports activities, or make a plan to transition publicly at school. You should "discuss" the bathroom issue (I used sarcastic quotation marks with "discuss," because it shouldn't really be a discussion—you simply need to let them know which bathrooms you feel the most comfortable using), and encourage them to create gender-neutral bathroom facilities if they do not already have them. You can also discuss (for realsies this time) how your school is going to provide resources and an expectation of respect and safety for you.

When your gender identity doesn't line up neatly with the box your doctor ticked when you were born, the pronouns that go along with that box may not fit you. Along similar lines, there may come a point that the name you were assigned at birth doesn't quite fit any longer, either. Sometimes coming out as trans, bi, gay, or lesbian can involve a complete reinvention of how you are in the world—including what people call you.

Your name is an integral part of your identity, not simply your gender identity. Though some people do not feel a name change necessary and are satisfied using their given name or a nickname, others find it important to claim a new name for themselves.

For people who wish to change their name, a legal name change is probably necessary at some point (see Legal Transition below), though asking others to use a new or different name, in the meantime, can be part of social transition as well.

You can find and access vocal coaching in your community to help tailor your vocal pitch to match your gender identity. Of course it is not a necessary part of social transition, but for some people, it can offer a sense of confidence and direction.

## LGBTW . . . The Name Thing

If you decide to change your name, strive to pick something that really fits you—something you love that you can feel comfortable with for the rest of your life.

Some ideas:

- Try the gender flip of your name; Allison could become Allister, Allen, or simply Al. William could become Willa, Wilma, or Willow . . .

- Go gender neutral; Andy, Bailey, Charlie . . .

- Respell or tweak your existing name; Dennis can become Denys, Ellie can be L. E.

- Pick a name from a hero, real or fictional, who has inspired you.

- You could get creative with other things that inspire you—perhaps a color, a plant, or a place—but use caution (see Other Tips, below). The more unusual the name, the more questions you will get about it from others.

- Pick a family name from an older relative.

- Scan places with big lists of names, like movie credits or books of baby names.

Once you've picked one, test it out for a bit before you commit. Ask a handful of your most-importants for some honest feedback or suggestions, practice writing it down and saying it out loud, start giving it out to the baristas at Starbucks. . . .

**Other tips:**

- Get comfortable with your name before you commit and advertise it—don't fall into the "I-know-I've-changed-my-name-seven-times-but-*this*-one-is-for-real!" trap.

- The "pop" in pop culture stands for "popular." And what is popular will change! So, think carefully before going with

"Katniss" or "McLovin"; they are your parents' "Ferris" or "Buffy" (go ask them, they'll explain).

- Don't legally change it for three to six months after starting to try it out.

- No tattoos until it's legal—tattooing a name on your body is always questionable, even if it's your own.

- Speaking of tattoos—remember, you will be sixty someday— you will have jobs, business cards, earn awards, and perhaps even have grandchildren. Shoot for a name that is going to last as well as represent you. What sounds cool at seventeen, may not at thirty . . .

- It takes time to get people on board, especially if they are used to calling you something different, but phrases like, "I prefer . . . ", and "My friends call me . . . " will help.

The deeper you get into your transition the more your natural voice, your natural style, and your natural "you" will come out, but in the early stages, finding a vocal and/or style mentor, such as a friend or perhaps a celebrity to emulate can make social transition feel less daunting. You could also search your app store for vocal training apps, specifically designed for people in transition, to help masculinize or feminize their voices.

We live in a very gendered society right now, and everything from shoes to sunglasses, backpacks to belts, and even your smartphone cover can look either masculine or feminine. These small, accessorizing changes, as well as the bigger-picture outfits you wear, will help you create a presentation of yourself that can accentuate the parts of yourself you want highlighted and diminish the parts you don't.

Many trans people are fortunate enough to have friends of their true gender. So enlisting a buddy or a bestie to help with shopping or even the loaning of clothes is a huge plus. Salespersons both in higher-end stores and in your funky, college-y, used shops can be great at helping you find a look that feels both fun and genuine.

**Tucking** refers to the process of hiding one's penis to create a more female-like crotch. Tucking is a way for many trans women to curb dysphoria, and is common during social transition.

Most women's clothing, even loose-fitting clothes to some extent, is not designed with extra room in the crotch, and whether you participate in medical transition or not, you may find that tucking your penis away helps complete your look.

You can tuck your penis and scrotum either up against your belly or back between your legs using tight-fitting underwear, garments called gaffs (super-tight fitting underwear designed to flatten and eliminate bulges), and/or sports or medical tape. (Did you see duct tape on that list? Do *not* use duct tape anywhere near your genitals!)

Your testicles can be inserted into your inguinal canal. This is where they go when it is very cold. Laying on your back it is possible to (carefully) rotate and (carefully) push them up into your abdomen. It can be uncomfortable at first, but should not hurt. They should easily come back out by (again carefully) pushing down on your abdomen just below your belly button until they dislodge.

Another perk of both testicle insertion and tighter-fitting garments is that keeping your testicles closer to your core body temperature will cause you to produce less testosterone! The reason testicles reside outside of our core body is that a slightly lower (typically 4 degrees or so) temperature is necessary for sperm and testosterone production, so a few extra degrees can often help slow down unwanted masculinization.

The process of tucking will become easier and more comfortable the more you practice, plus if you do start HRT, your external genitalia will reduce in size and erections will become less frequent, making the processes even easier.

**Stuffing** refers to using materials such as padding, bras, and prosthetic breasts called breastforms that can help create cleavage for MTF people who are socially transitioning.

**Packing** is the FTM version—using materials such as a rolled-up sock, secured with a safety pin or jockstrap, or commercially bought prosthetics, called packers, made of silicone (some can even make it so you can pee while standing) to help create a male-like bulge in your crotch.

## LGBTW . . . Cautions About Tucking

Tape can be irritating, so use medical or sports tape, which is easier on the skin, and if any irritation develops, stop. The benefit of a clean line is not worth the pain.

Similarly if you have difficulty tucking your testicles into your inguinal canals, then do not force them. If there is pain or too much needed effort, then you are either doing it incorrectly or it simply won't work for your body.

Tucking your penis between your legs and leaving your testicles on either side (and hidden by your thighs) should work just fine—just avoid bicycles, jogging, and sitting down too quickly!

There is a slight increased chance of urinary tract infections from tucking as this can place your urethra closer to your anus, so keep it clean (wipe front to back), talk to your doctor, and drink cranberry juice—it is your friend.

Don't tuck 24/7. In fact, don't tuck for more than eight to twelve hours at a time, and of course if anything goes wrong, see a doctor.

## LGBTW . . . Peeing

Though peeing while standing can be considered a great freedom by some people with penises, it is not necessarily all it is cracked up to be. It can be easier in some situations (and there are always those stories about the joys of writing one's name in the snow), but you do have to concentrate. Like, the whole, entire time.

Though many places now have gender-neutral bathrooms, there are still plenty of public restrooms designated "men's" or "women's."

Some trans guys can feel very self-conscious in the men's restroom, but there really is not much need. Men's rooms are different than women's.

Primarily, people do not tend to do much talking and even less looking around. In fact, turning the head while at the urinal is a huge no-no in men's bathrooms (so is using your phone, gross).

Generally, men's room etiquette says: Get in. Do your stuff. Get out.

Other details that might help:

- When possible, leave an unoccupied urinal between you and the next person (I know, I know . . . just do it).

- Aim.

- Again, no talking (except possibly at the sink, and even then that is typically limited to, "Hey," "What's up?" and "Have a good one."). Also, no singing, whistling, or humming. Because, awkward.

- Stand tall, keep your stance narrow, pick a point on the wall, and focus.

- Aim.

And there is never shame in picking a stall for some added privacy.

There is also no shame in sitting to pee. (1) Most people are going to go number one if they are already down there going number two anyway, and (2) *Zero* people are going to be standing outside the stall door listening to verify what you are doing (see above re: get in / get out), and (3) you can actually relax! (But also see above re: no phones.)

If you are new to peeing standing up, and/or are using a prosthesis that will allow you to pee standing, practice at home before taking your show on the road. If you do have some splash issue (which everyone with a penis does from time to time), after washing your hands, "accidentally" splash a bit of water on the fronts of your trousers and shirt—people (if they even notice) will assume it was a sink issue!

**Binding** refers to the process of flattening one's breasts in order to create a more male-like chest. Chest binding is a way for many trans men to curb dysphoria, and is common during social transition.

While binding with common household items such as Ace bandages and tape can be less expensive, they aren't made for binding, and can cause harm such as rashes, scarring, and restricted breathing.

Sports bras or commercially purchased binders are a safer and more effective way to go. There are two types of binders: short ones and long ones. The shorter ones end at your waist. The longer ones go several inches past your waist, and can be tucked into pants, creating a leaner look.

Free and discounted, donated bras and binders can be found online via donation at websites like www.transactiveonline.org. You can also donate your used ones and help someone else out as well.

The process of binding will become easier and more comfortable the more you practice, plus if you do start HRT, your breasts will reduce in size, making the process even easier.

---

### LGBTW . . . Cautions About Binding

Binders and sports bras may not breathe well and can be hot, sweaty, and uncomfortable. To minimize skin irritation and soreness, try wearing undershirts, using body powder, and keeping your binder as clean as possible.

Be safe. Any methods of binding can be uncomfortable, or even painful, but if too small or tight, it can restrict your movement and even your breathing. Buy the binder that fits the body you have, not the body you want to have, and don't cinch it up like you're in a Jane Austen novel. If it hurts, cuts your skin, or prevents you from breathing, it is too tight.

Don't bind 24/7. In fact, don't bind for more than eight to twelve hours at a time, and of course if anything goes wrong, see a doctor.

---

Social transition may put a strain on your family. Even if you are fortunate enough to have folks that fully support you, it may still be hard on them. Do what you can to make it easier. Be appreciative. Be patient. Be kind.

Some people choose to move in or live temporarily with extended family or friends during social and medical transition. This can help with social transition, especially if you choose to change schools.

But be sure to spend time and stay in contact with supportive parents and siblings. Don't underestimate how much they will miss you and will want to be an active part of your transition.

---

### LGBTW . . . Social Media

Compared to other identifying populations, there just are not that many trans people. At least at this point, researchers are estimating that about a tenth of the number of Americans who identify as lesbian, gay, or bisexual identify as trans.[1] It can be very difficult outside of major, metropolitan cities to form communities based on proximity, but connecting people who are spread across vast geographies into a single community is exactly the sort of problem the Internet was designed to solve!

People being able to experience other peoples' experience through media helps humanize us all and remove some of the politics from our perceptions. This is why television was so helpful in terms of the civil rights movements that began in the 1960s. In the 1990s, the Web went mainstream, and the more visible gay people became in the culture and in straight people's day-to-day lives, the more accepting the world became. Now, social media is the tool for the trans movement.

For L, G, B, and T people, online interaction can offer an excellent third space, apart from being closeted or stealth, to being out. During early social transition, it can also be a nice way to test out a new way of being social.

Trans and other queer people can use social media as a space to share stories and experience, to connect with others, find support and guidance, and document collective history.

We know now that visibility and affirmation can be vital to acceptance and even survival. Sites like Facebook, Instagram, Tumblr, Twitter, and YouTube can help. There are loads of inspiring YouTube vlogs and Facebook groups, Reddit conversations, and dozens and dozens of memes and sites to help explain the admittedly complicated Rubik's Cube that is sex, gender, orientation, and expression (see chapters 6 and 7).

TrevorSpace and Distinc.tt are social networking sites for GLBTQ youth (ages thirteen to twenty-four) and their friends and allies that may not feel as public as Instagram or Snapchat. The app GayBFF uses an interface that is similar to dating apps to help LGBT people and their allies find friends, social outlets, and community without the pressure or expectation of love, sex, and romance, matching users with like-minded individuals with the potential to become friends.

Even though the larger GLBTQ community has seen progress on legal and social acceptance, the rates of depression, loneliness, and substance abuse when individual queer people feel alone and alienated are still a huge problem, and social media can be a very validating and community-building force for cultural change. As young gay, lesbian, and bisexual people continue to come out via social media, more and more gay and lesbian adults, celebrities, and professional sports figures are finding the inspiration and voice to come out at later ages as well.

For trans kids this can be different. Someone who identifies as gay or lesbian will likely still be doing so in ten, twenty, or forty years. That is not necessarily the same for trans people. Some people choose to shut down previous profiles and start from zero after transitioning, choosing to live their life (both analog and digital) as their real/true gender. Others are OK updating previous profiles and identifying publicly as trans on their social media. The choice whether or not to tie your new name/gender identity to the one assigned to you at birth via social media is a big choice that may be hard to un-choose. So consider your process, and your end goals and philosophies around trans identity, before plugging in. The Internet is *forever*.

Online life aside, for some transgender people, once they have begun to socially transition, the next step of learning how to be who they are may also include the option of physically changing their bodies to better align their identity with their physical sex.

This may or may not be a necessary part of your plan for yourself, but for every trans person, physically transitioning or changing gender or sex is a big decision—because many of those changes are permanent.

## Medical Transition

It is important to note that some transgender people want their authentic gender identity to be recognized without hormones or surgery. Others may lack the access or resources to such medical care. There is no right or wrong way to transition, and a transgender identity is not dependent on medical procedures.

But for those who can and do utilize medical procedures in their transition, the two primary ways people do this are through hormone replacement therapy (HRT) and surgery.

The World Professional Association for Transgender Health (WPATH), outlined standards of care for people who are accessing medical transition.[2]

The first stage of this is, typically, meeting with a mental health professional for a diagnosis and psychotherapy. The current version of WPATH's standards recommends that mental health professionals provide a series of

---

### LGBTW . . . Gender Confirmation Surgery

Though gender confirmation surgery is also known as gender reassignment, gender replacement, or sex reassignment surgery, the term "sex reassignment surgery" is falling out of use both as an acknowledgment that the process is about gender not sex, and as an emphasis on the treatment and integration of the mind and body, not simply the medical procedure itself.

---

letters prior to medical transition. A letter from a therapist, usually with a diagnosis of gender dysphoria, is required to allow a person to begin hormone therapy with a medical doctor.

You do *not* need to change doctors if you have a doctor or pediatrician whom you have seen for several years and/or feel comfortable with. Your doctor (if they are not comfortable or well-versed with gender issues) can work together with other medical and mental health professionals who are more specialized in gender-specific care.

The next stage is referred to as "The Real-Life Experience," during which individuals seeking hormonal and other treatments are encouraged (and expected) to socially transition to their true gender role if they have not done so already.

The final stage involves the actual, physical surgeries. At this point a second letter is required for the top surgeries, and two additional letters are needed for the bottom surgeries, to verify that the person is both eligible and ready for gender reassignment.

## Hormone Replacement Therapy (HRT)

Some people believe you have to wait until eighteen to begin HRT, but you do not. Having your parents and/or a talk therapist advocate for you can help.

Many trans people have waited (sometimes long) periods of time before making permanent changes, and there are benefits to waiting. These benefits include having more time to plan strategies and budgets and to form and solidify support systems. Additionally, as time passes better/more/easier interventions may become possible and available.

However slow or fast your transition of your physical body is, your gender identity is yours, and waiting doesn't take away anything from who you are.

If your doctor tries to talk you into delaying puberty rather than transition, this is likely because they want you to have the opportunity to hit the pause button on the effects of natal puberty, take time to explore your feelings and options, and give you and your family time to plan what happens next (and possibly to make themselves feel more comfortable).

---

## LGBTW . . . Blockers

Sometimes doctors prescribe medications to tweens and teens that halt the puberty hormones that masculinize or feminize a body with secondary sex characteristics. These are called puberty blockers. Studies show that trans youth who undergo treatments to delay puberty showed improved, long-term psychological well-being.[3]

Suppressing your puberty by using hormone blockers can give you the opportunity to develop into a young adult without developing unwanted sex characteristics like voice changes or hair growth that can be difficult to undo.

Blockers wont take away what puberty changes have already occurred, but they will (temporarily) stop the progression of hormone-induced biological changes. Plus, they are reversible, and allow trans youth to start the process of transitioning at younger ages than previous generations have been able to.

Historically, treatment of transgender people didn't start until they reached adulthood, finished puberty, and had developed physical changes that were irreversible and potentially distressing.

The Endocrine Society of Transgender Persons' guidelines[4] suggest starting puberty blockers for transgender children around ten or eleven years old for (natal) girls and eleven or twelve years old for (natal) boys. This allows for more time to get clearer about decisions and can prevent increased dysphoria that can accompany puberty for trans youth.

When and if to start cross-sex hormones depends on each person's stability, readiness, and confidence, in their gender identity.

Though The Endocrine Society's guidelines also recommend beginning HRT at age sixteen (because of the impact that delaying puberty for too long can have on physical, emotional, and social development), more and more trans kids are starting hormones at thirteen or fourteen if their doctors, therapists, and families agree that they are mentally and emotionally prepared.

This generation is the first to have the option to start taking hormones so young, and more research is needed on blockers' impact on body and brain development (including cancer and fertility issues), but at the time of this writing, many doctors are in agreement that the benefits appear to be outweighing the risks.[5]

When you have discussed this with your family and therapist, and you feel certain and ready to start HRT, if your doctor *still* tries to talk you into waiting to transition, stay vocal, take the initiative, and insist on starting HRT and/or seeking a second opinion.

There are three different ways to medically get hormones: injections, pills, or topical solutions.

Injection is the most effective way to receive your hormones because it can be injected straight into the muscle (intramuscularly, or IM) or under the skin (subcutaneously or SQ) and absorbed quickly. Injections can be cumbersome and some people are squicked out by having to get (or give themselves) injections.

Pills (either swallowed or dissolved under the tongue) are the second most effective. They are easier than injections, though can be slower in terms of effect. The frequency and dosage is different person-to-person.

Topical solutions, such as creams, lotions, or patches, are the least effective method, though beneficial if you want to start your HRT slowly and more gently.

The delivery method is up to each, individual person, and the results will also vary. Effects of hormones can be felt sooner for some people than others depending on your physical makeup and dosages, but within a month or two most people report a sense that their insides and outsides feel more in alignment, and that sense of gender dysphoria is diminished (which is one of the biggest benefits of HRT).

*For FTM trans people*[6]

Androgens like testosterone (generally called "T"), dehydroepiandrosterone (DHEA), and dihydrotestosterone (DHT) can be given to help develop secondary, male characteristics such as muscle development and body hair, as well as suppressing natural estrogen production and preventing/ending menstruation.

For some FTM minors, it may be a good idea to choose to delay puberty with puberty blockers in combination with low doses of testosterone. As boys typically develop later than girls, human growth hormone can be added to the testosterone treatment throughout puberty to help reach average male height and build.

Hair growth aids can be prescribed to encourage facial and body hair.

***Effects of androgens:***[7]   Within the first six months after starting androgens, your sex drive can increase (sometimes in surprisingly noticeable ways), and the frequency, intensity, and duration of feeling horny may all go up. Your clitoris may grow slightly thicker or longer, as will the hair on your arms and legs. Hair may also grow on your chest, back, and belly. Vaginal dryness and increased muscle mass and upper body strength are common, as is a shifting of body fat (from hips to waist), creating a more masculine body shape. Your menstrual periods will likely stop during this time.

After about a year you may begin to grow hair on your face and lose some from your head (though both full beard growth and male-pattern baldness can take several years to develop).

*For MTF trans people*[8]

Estrogen (to help maintain the levels that genetic or natal women produce naturally) and anti-androgens (which stop and/or reverse the masculinizing effects of male hormones such as testosterone) can help change musculature, skin and fat distribution, and diminish body hair.

Sometimes a progestogen is also added to the mix to support, supplement, or replace estrogen if needed.

Topical creams or laser treatments can help with hair removal for those who may have started puberty before transitioning.

Silicone can be implanted into breasts, buttocks, and faces to provide more curves and definition for MTF people. Most plastic surgeons agree that these processes are safest when used as enclosed implants of medical-grade silicone.

*Effects of estrogen/anti-androgens:*[9] Within the first six months after starting estrogen a decrease in sex drive is generally noted, including fewer (and softer) spontaneous erections. Your skin may become softer and a decrease in muscle mass is common, as is a shifting of body fat (from waist to hips), creating a more stereotypically feminine body shape. Erections may decrease or completely stop during this time, as can your ability to produce sperm and semen (you may still ejaculate, and the fluid may still contain active sperm, though the fluid will become clearer and less thick).

Over the next year or two you can notice a decrease in body hair growth. Breast and nipples can become larger while your penis and testicles may reduce in size (though this can happen over a period of several years).

The interventions that are available change rapidly as the science and culture evolve. If/when you find yourself considering *any* sort of medical intervention, this writer suggests

- Doing diligent research.

- Talking to your doctor about your findings.

- Forming a realistic plan that works for you.

- Participating in talk therapy with someone both knowledgeable and comfortable with the subject of gender.

- Surrounding yourself with supportive people.

*Other impacts of HRT*

HRT begins to create changes in a person's body from the inside out, by the addition of opposite sex hormones into one's body and/or the stopping or subtraction of the hormones made naturally by the body one was born into. Both internally and externally, these new hormones can change your experience in various ways.

**HRT can impact physical health.** There are loads of positive physical changes when trans people begin HRT; however there can be negative, physical side effects as well.

The hormones associated with FTM transition can increase the risk of heart disease (including heart attack), stroke, and diabetes. The risks are greater if you smoke, are overweight, or have a family history of heart disease or diabetes.[10]

The hormones associated with MTF transition can increase your risk of heart disease (including heart attack), blood clots, diabetes, and other issues including gallstones. Increases in headaches, nausea, and blood pressure are also associated with estrogen. Anti-androgens are known for contributing to skin rashes and changes in heart rhythm for some people.[11]

Minimizing contributing factors like not smoking (which is a great idea for everyone), staying fit and active, and eating well are things you can do to reduce risk, as well as staying in communication with your health professionals about your specific needs and potential risks.

***HRT can impact mental health.*** There are often positive emotional changes from reduced gender dysphoria after trans people begin HRT; however there can be negative, emotional side effects as well.

For some FTM trans people, the increased testosterone can result in increased frustration, irritability, and even anger. Increases in sex drive are often noted by FTM trans people who begin testosterone, which doesn't necessarily sound like a bad thing, but the changes can be overwhelming for some and, for others, the wanting to have more sex can lead to feelings of loneliness (especially if you are not having sex with anyone). For trans men who are also diagnosed with bipolar or any of the schizoaffective disorders, testosterone can sometimes make their symptoms worse.[12]

MTF people on hormones often cite a broader range of emotion and emotional expression as well—not only feeling more "feels," but also wanting to tell others about them. Some cite irritability, but the most common side effect is the expression of sadness—not necessarily more sadness than usual, but more crying when you are sad. The tears can come on suddenly and then can just keep coming for a while . . . this can be about legitimate sad things in the news or your personal life or those commercials about all the sick animals, or can be about happy things like flash mobs or those commercials about the soldiers who come back and surprise their families. The feels are for understandable reasons, but the volume can be turned up and this can be confusing and uncomfortable—especially if you were not a big crier before HRT.

For your emotional health, stay in communication with your doctors, work to find the dosage and administration method (patches, pills, or injections) that work best for your own, unique chemistry, and make sure to have people both personally and professionally you can talk to.

***HRT can impact sexual health.*** Everyone's experience will vary once they begin HRT. Though changes (good and bad) in sex drive are common, changes relating to the experience of and interest in sex can occur as well.

Different than the typical increase in libido for trans men, trans women often notice a lowered sex drive. Like the increase mentioned above, this is not necessarily a good or bad thing, but for some it is a notable change that often rebalances itself over time.

Some transgender people (both trans men and trans women) can experience a change in their sexual orientation after they begin HRT. Many who were attracted to women prior to transitioning may remain attracted to women after they begin HRT, though others might find themselves attracted to men instead (or sometimes in addition).

People's experience of their own orgasm can change as well after HRT. Trans men may experience a more focused or concentrated feel to their orgasms that they may find easier to have, while trans women may notice a broader, whole-body-feel to theirs that may take longer to achieve than they did prior to transitioning.

All of these experiences are 100 percent normative and 100 percent OK, though if any of them become troubling or difficult to deal with, seeking out information, resources, and professional support is a very good thing.

***HRT can impact social health.*** Though interpersonal factors such as self-esteem and confidence can be improved by beginning HRT, there are social challenges that can come after transition begins.

While it is possible for some to choose to stay closeted or to go stealth after beginning HRT, for others the changes that hormones can cause can be quite visible, such as breast growth or facial hair and voice changes. Being visibly trans in a transphobic society has social risks.

In addition to the extra work, and the rejection (which trans people share with gay, lesbian, and bi people), there is also the potential violence (which they also share); however people who identify as trans are almost twice (1.58 times) as likely to experience injuries from hate violence than the rest of the LGBT community.[13]

But apart from the things you share with the rest of the GLBT population, as a trans person, the act of disclosure can put you in the position of becoming a walking wiki for the entire trans phenomenon, having to field questions ranging from the kinda-insulting ("I feel like I shouldn't be attracted to you, but I am" / "I would have never known you were trans") to the absolutely ridiculous ("If I'm attracted to you does that make me gay?") to the super rude ("Are you pre-op?" / "What do your genitals look like?").

Many relationships change (in good ways and in bad) as a person transitions. An FTM person may notice, for example that being their siblings' brother looks and feels different than it did when they were their siblings' sister. Some dating and romantic relationships survive when one member transitions and the other does not. And a MTF person who stays with her female partner after transitioning may find being in a relationship with another woman quite different than it was when their bodies were different.

Proactively anticipating some of these reactions from people you may encounter and keeping your level of personal safety as high as possible can help, as well as creating a supportive community and participating in LGBTQ activism both locally and nationally.

## LGBTW . . . Patience

The process of medical transition can be long, complicated, and expensive. There are people who prey on transgender people who don't have the patience, insurance, ego strength, or financial resources to make this easier.

There are underground hormones often promoted online. They do not work and are extremely dangerous. Whether pills or injections to quickly increase muscle mass, lose weight, or develop breast tissue, you can waste you time and money and can make yourself sick—maybe even dead.

People can be tempted to go online for hormones because of biased or unhelpful insurance plans, insurance that may have to be accessed through unsupportive parents, or a general lack of gender-specific care in their area. *But*:

- Using underground hormones can interfere with any legitimate hormone therapy you are doing or may do in the future.

- The dosage can be hard to define, and deadly to experiment with.

- Underground needles and syringes for injections can be unsanitary—raising the risk of contracting both HIV and viral hepatitis.

- It is impossible to verify that what you are paying for or taking are actually the hormones you are seeking.

Liquid or loose (not enclosed) silicone injections are sometimes advertised to trans women by people referred to as "pumpers." Although many pumpers say they have been previously trained as nurses, most have no medical training and are not licensed to perform surgical procedures. Like those who perform back-alley abortions, they often operate in rooms that are not sterile, using industrial-grade silicone (the kind used for planes and automobiles) or medical-grade that has been cut with cooking or baby oils—increasing the risk of infection. Regardless of the silicone used, when injected loosely, it can migrate, solidify, cause permanent disfiguration, and sometimes enter the bloodstream. This is highly dangerous and should be avoided. If you do not believe me, Google it—it's chilling. If you desire silicone, it is best to wait until you have fully grown into your adult body and are in a financial position to afford legitimate, closed implants from a trained plastic surgeon.

Do not let people prey on your insecurities or need. Like puberty, transition is not easy or quick. It's not supposed to be. Do not go into any part of this trying to convince yourself that it will be either easy or quick, and be *very* suspicious of anyone who tries to convince you otherwise. There are no magic wands, genie lamps, or time machines. These processes may involve waiting and/or saving up for quite a while—perhaps years. And that is OK.

Transition takes planning, and insight, support, and information. That is part of why it is such a serious and important process.

It also takes a strong person to transition. That is part of why you are holding this book in your hand. So,

- Be strong.

- Remember that the mental and emotional changes are just as important as the outside stuff.

- Concentrate on loving and learning about yourself as you grow and change.

- Take your time!

## The Real-Life Experience

Sometimes known as the Real-Life Test (or simply RLE), The Real-Life Experience usually requires candidates for gender replacement surgery to live full-time (sometimes for as long as a year) as their real gender. The purpose of an RLE is to confirm that you are able to function successfully as a member of your accurate gender in society, as well as to make sure that you are ready to live as that gender for the rest of your life.

An RLE used to be a requirement of some physicians before performing medical transition, sometimes before legal transition, and occasionally before hormone replacement therapy (HRT). Though, the most recent edition of the standards has removed specific parameters for the RLE, but state that the individual should be living full-time in their preferred gender role continuously for the duration of the RLE.[14]

Changing your name as well as your gender markers and documentation in places such as school and work can help you document the experience of people other than family, friends, and your therapist knowing you in your accurate gender. This can also be considered evidence that you have completed your Real-Life Experience.[15]

## Gender Confirmation Surgery

So after you've socially transitioned, begun HRT, and completed your Real-Life Experience, surgery may be the next step for you.

The physical surgeries themselves are broken down both by gender (men transitioning to women or women transitioning to men) and geography ("top" surgeries, above the waist and "bottom" surgeries, below).

Male to female genital surgery is, typically, less expensive and less invasive than female to male surgery.

For MTF people the Top surgeries include:

- Augmentation mammoplasty in which the breasts are enlarged.

- Men transitioning to women can also have plastic surgery to "feminize" their faces and necks, including work on their eyes, noses, brows, chins, and hairlines, and can have their Adam's apple shaved down so it is less prominent.

For MTF people the Bottom surgeries include:

- Castration, in which the testicles and most of the penis are removed and the urethra is cut shorter.

- Vaginoplasty, in which some of the skin is used to fashion a largely functional vagina.

- A "neoclitoris" that allows sensation can be created from parts of the penis.

Female to male genital surgery is more difficult, more costly, and generally more invasive than male to female surgery. This is why fewer trans men choose to have genital reconstruction surgery than trans women.

For FTM people the Top surgeries include:

- Removing breasts (male chest reconstruction).

For FTM people the Bottom surgeries include:

- Hysterectomy, in which the uterus and ovaries are removed.

- Metoidioplasty, in which the clitoris is released and made to appear longer, can allow for sexual sensation. This can sometimes be combined with a urethral extension to allow trans guys to pee while standing.

- Scrotoplasty, in which the labia majora are used to form a scrotum. A process called fat grafting (or implanting prosthetic testicles) can be done for realism.

A fully functioning penis cannot be surgically created at this point, but genitals (and other tissues) can be manipulated surgically to resemble a penis in many ways. Many trans men can eventually even pee standing up, and there are procedures (such as permanent, bendable rods and inflatable implants with pumps disguised as testicles) that can facilitate erections.

The interventions that are available change rapidly as the science and culture evolve. If/when you find yourself considering *any* sort of medical intervention, this writer suggests

- Getting clear about what results you want.

- Doing diligent research.

- Talking to your doctor about your findings.

- Forming a realistic plan that works for you.

- Participating in talk therapy with someone both knowledgeable and comfortable with the subject of gender.

- Surrounding yourself with supportive people.

While not everyone who is trans will transition medically, if you are interested in exploring this option, take some time to research medical professionals in your area. You may live in areas with limited options, but it is important to explore your options. For more information on health care and providers, you can visit the Gay & Lesbian Medical Association (GLMA.org) or check out HRC's transgender resources (HRC.org).

The idea that everyone who is trans *needs* to have HRT or surgery is shifting. While many people feel internal and/or external pressure to have their body conform to their gender, there is no "correct" path to take. As noted elsewhere, the important thing is to be true to oneself.

## Legal Transition

The final piece of transition is legal transition. This involves updating the name and gender markers on your school and state IDs and state-issued driver's license. Social Security cards, birth certificates, and passports can also be changed.

Changing your name and gender on your official documents can help:

- Avoid harassment and discrimination.

- Make accessing education, jobs, health care, voting, traveling, and public and financial services easier.

This doesn't mean you need to come out to the whole world—only those who are in charge of sorting out your documentations.

### Changing Your Name

For many transgender people, securing a legal name change is an important step toward making their legal identities match their lived experience.

Officially changing your name can make the rest of these legal changes easier. This should be a relatively simple process (married people do it every day), which generally involves a court date, but not necessarily an attorney.

Many states allow you to use whatever name you wish, so long as you are consistent. If you're under eighteen, however, you will need parental or guardian consent.

Some people choose to wait until adulthood to change their name officially, though the benefits of doing this in your teens include having your name be accurate on school records, including your diploma and social media.

The Standards of Care from the World Professional Association for Transgender Health (WPATH)[16] encouraged the US State Department and the Social Security Administration to change their policies for updating passports and Social Security cards to require only a doctor's letter explaining that you *must* use your new name as part of your medical treatment and asking that any and all who read that letter help in this matter.

In most cases you can update your name and gender at the same time. You should not be asked any inappropriate or super-invasive questions about your transition or medical history to make this happen, and if you are, you may want that attorney to help you after all.

Then, get as many IDs as you can in your new name. Go to the library and get a new library card. Join a gym and other clubs or associations that issue ID membership cards. Get bills sent to your house with your new name. Open a checking account. Get a debit card. Thinking of as many places as possible where you can create your new public identity as possible will make getting other, accurate government IDs easier.

### Changing Your State IDs and Driver's License

The process of changing your gender on your driver's license varies state by state. For more information, including your state's policies, visit LambdaLegal.org or TransEquality.org.

### Changing Your Social Security Card

Though your gender is not actually listed on your Social Security card, the Social Security Administration (SSA) tracks gender as part of your electronic record.

According to the SSA policies,[17] you can now change your gender with the SSA with any of the following: an accurate birth certificate or passport, a court order, or a letter from your doctor like the one mentioned above.

### Changing Your Birth Certificate

Birth certificate policies can also vary state by state. Birth certificates are considered vital records, so the process is often more complicated and generally requires a court order. Some states require proof of gender reassignment, three states will not alter birth certificates to reflect someone's correct sex (Kansas, Idaho, and Ohio), and one state currently (2017!) has statutes in place that actually forbid the correction of sex designations on birth certificates for trans people (hint: it rhymes with Tennessee).[18]

### Changing Your Passport

For this, you will likely need a letter from your doctor (including their name, address, information about their medical license) as a statement that you have received clinical treatment to facilitate gender reassignment. This can mean anything from simply living as your correct gender to taking hormones or having surgery.

People whose transitions are not yet completed can request a limited, two-year passport along with a letter from your doctor explaining that you are still in the transition process.[19]

For more information, including sample physician letters, visit LambdaLegal.org or TransEquality.org.

This process can be difficult, especially if you are a minor with an unsupportive family or only partially transitioned. However, there are laws in place for discrimination, so no need to be scared. You can seek legal assistance from the Transgender Legal Defense & Education Fund, Lambda Legal, or the Transgender Law Center.

For people who feel distressed by the differences between their identity and their physical body, social, medical, and/or legal transition, can provide some harmony, a sense of integrity, and other positive mental changes.

That being said, support through this process is *very* important, and no one should have to go through this process alone. Supportive friends, family, medical professionals, and counseling make a huge difference in how each particular person navigates and adjusts to their transition.

Transitioning is courageous and beautiful, because it is such an important choice. These changes should not be taken lightly. Ask questions. Seek out guidance and mentors. Understand details and weigh options. Use resources. And never regret anything you do to make your life and your body more yours.

---

### LGBTW . . . pride (with a lower-case p)

Don't forget to celebrate! Spending time and energy figuring out who you are, and then working to manifest that in the world, is a *huge* accomplishment. Be proud and honor yourself—some trans people even pick a transition date, and celebrate it, like a birthday.

---

# PASSING

Passing is a somewhat-problematic concept that is about being accepted as / believed to be in your chosen gender without your trans status being known, discovered, or divulged. A passing trans person's gender is not evident or obvious simply by looking at them.

"Stealth" and "woodworking" are also terms for a trans person who does not show up as (or may not even identify publicly as) trans. A trans person "living stealth" theoretically shows up as indistinguishable from a cis person.

The opposite of passing or living stealth is being "clocked" or "read," meaning they have been recognized as a transgender person.

Passing is a controversial term for some people, because it conjures the idea of "trying," "playing at," or "acting a part." Passing can sound like an effortful covering up of a person's "transness" or gender differences—not just through their appearance, but by creating fictions about their past, and hiding (or actively lying about) their relationship to the gender they were identified as at birth.

This would be considered in opposition to simply being who you are (both inside and out) in a genuine and transparent way, *and* without other people being or becoming aware of your trans status or history.

There are other terms that may be less loaded, like "blending" or "being transparent," but the bottom line is there is no shame in making your inside experience match your outer appearance, in being the most You you can be or in doing whatever you need to for your own personal sense of peace and happiness.

**There are benefits to passing/blending.**

Passing/blending can

- allow open movement without fear of harassment, discrimination, and violence.

- facilitate securing employment, housing, and socialization.

- provide a sense of accomplishment.

- help you feel more physically protected, mentally congruent, and emotionally comfortable.

**There are problems associated with passing/blending.**

There is a myth that all trans people can pass if they try hard enough—if they take enough hormones, if they get enough surgery, and put enough energy into adopting the other gender completely. Some trans people struggle with both self-acceptance and self-respect, and can feel a lot of societal pressure to pass—feeling like a failure if they do not.

The difficulty of becoming passable depends on several factors, all of which vary greatly, including:

- facial and bone structure.

- individual responses to hormone therapy.

- Some trans people's body development, shape, and size may defy social or medical interventions.

- the costs and degree of surgical procedures.

- the coverage or presence of insurance plans.

- Fully transitioning can involve multiple medical interventions. Trans people who are dependent on others, who are unsupported by family, who are homeless, in jobs with certain insurance structures or areas with fewer resources may not have access to high-quality transition-related health care.

- the impact of geography, local laws, and the Internet on how much control one has over their own documentation.

- US states' differing rules around altering legal documents, and the Internet itself, can make erasing a past difficult, if not impossible.

Some people associate passing as the trans equivalent to staying in / going back into the closet. The idea being that, if you are living as a trans girl in stealth mode that you have a secret you're not sharing or are secretly living as a girl, or that if you are "passing as" a boy, then you are not *truly* a boy.

But: Trans boys are *not* girls in disguise, regardless of whether people know the gender that was assigned to them at birth—trans boys are *men*.

Trans girls are *not* boys in a costume—trans girls are *women*.

Period.

Underlined.

The legitimacy of your relationship to your own identity does not change because the friend you are having lunch with (who knows) goes to the bathroom, leaving you alone at the table with the waiter (who doesn't).

Plus, the trans equivalent of being out is being open and honest about one's gender identity. So anytime you are identifying yourself with the gender you know yourself to be, you are out, and showing those around you how good you are at being you.

Do not let anyone tell you that introducing yourself to everyone you meet with, "Hey, I'm trans!" needs to be a necessary part of being trans. Cis people don't have to announce such things. Gay people don't need to describe kissing people of the opposite sex before coming out as proof they are *actually* gay.

Stating, implying, or acting as though trans people who do not disclose their trans status are somehow not *really* trans is called stealth-shaming. And it's not OK.

In many ways, the opposite is true; transitioning to the point in which your dress, demeanor, and deeds allow you to confidently embody the gender to which you always knew you belonged is similar to a gay person coming out and saying "this is who I am / who I was meant to be."

A gay person having the insight and ego strength to acknowledge and identify their true orientation in a clear and shame-free way isn't seen as a bad thing—so having pride in accessing your true gender in a legitimate and effortful way (whether it is obvious to others or not) shouldn't be either.

That being said:

Being truly you, and making your outward appearance as congruent with that as possible, does *not* mean that you must ditch any of your trans friends, abandon your past, or orphan yourself or your history in any way.

Who you were and where you came from are part of your journey, and have contributed to making you *The You* you are now, and will contribute to *The You* you will grow to be.

You don't need to wear an "I'm trans, ask me how!" T-shirt, mention your birth gender in your yearbook photos, or fill your Instagram feed with TBT photos of your pre-transition sex or gender—*but*, being closeted about your past and your transition can lead you to being closeted about who you currently are and someday will be.

You also don't need to paint yourself into any corners in which you can't be authentically who you are, in which you have to go back to feeling like you are living a lie or like you can't share your history with people.

Be safe, and choose carefully whom you share your story and status with. Privacy is important (sometimes safer and smarter and even empowering), but being truthful with friends, supportive family members, partners, and doctors (even if you are blending full time) is important too.

## LGBTW . . . Privilege

Privilege is about the advantages people get because they belong to certain sets of the population. These sets include sex and gender, but also race (the biologically inherited traits from your physical heritage), ethnicity (the culturally inherited characteristics we get from our families and the places from which they come), and socioeconomic status.

Typically, the more white, male, cis, and wealthy you are, the more privilege you have and the more entitlement you feel.

The more privilege you have, the more you see yourself reflected in movies, commercials, song lyrics, and other media, the more you can read about people like yourself in history books and popular fiction, and the less you have to worry about safety and oppression in laws, education, and the job market or being targeted or attacked either online or in real life (IRL).

Passing Privilege is the belief that trans people who "pass" enjoy greater acceptance in society. This is similar to Bi Privilege, with the idea being that they can go through their day to day existence looking either straight (if you're bi) or cis (if you're trans), thereby experiencing more positive and/or less negative interactions than their gay or trans peers.

If you pass, live stealth, or become blended or transparent, you have successfully adapted to the gender you subscribe to, and other people may not know that you transitioned at all. Your choice then, to identify, come out, or be out as trans, is still exactly that—your choice.

Passing/blending can be showing others exactly who you were meant to be from the beginning, leading with the parts of you that were hidden and unsurfaced, successfully presenting (and being accepted as) your chosen gender—whether or not you keep the fact that you are trans to yourself.

- It is not the same as being gay (or bi or lesbian) and closeted if you are not out as trans.

- It's OK for the rules to be a bit different.

- Being gay and being trans *are* different (yes, they are all included in the GLBT initialism, but the L, G, and B are sexual orientations, the T is not).

If someone fully integrates and lives in their chosen gender do they have to ID as trans? Can there be a point at which they simply identify as a man or a woman? Does it have to come down to being either trans or cis? These are questions that each person has to answer for themselves,

## PART FOUR
# "LET'S HAVE A KIKI"

Dating is meant to be fun. That being said, in a culture of friend requests, when most people have fewer IRL connections than online ones and a tendency to text more than talk, dating can also be stressful and confusing for gay, straight, bi, and trans people.

Some people blame social media for this generalized/generational loss of dating skill, but most of you reading this book may simply never have had the opportunity to form those skills in the first place. Besides, while living in an insta-age of fleeting contacts, waiting for the next upgrade and vague "We-should-totally-get-togethers" and "Wanna hang-outs?"—it is *not* weird that the progressive, sometimes-coded and complicated process of dating has fallen to the wayside.

A dick pic has replaced flowers and chocolate, and dinner and a movie has been replaced by Netflix and chill (which is itself just code for let's *not* watch the movie . . . ). Hookup apps now pose as dating apps—simultaneously making flirting and sweet/awkward negotiation obsolete *and* creating a polarized choice between being "friends" or being a hookup. Swipe left or swipe right . . . no one knows how to date any more. Relationships are labeled "It's complicated"? Absolutely.

But dating does not actually have to be all that complicated.

## CHAPTER FOURTEEN
# DATING

## Before a Date

- Plan it—there is something to be said for the romance of spontaneity, but showing someone you have been thinking about them can be much more powerful (plus, if you wait until the last minute to ask someone out, you run the risk of communicating to them that you are assuming they have nothing better to do than sit around waiting for your text).

- Dates, especially the first one, do not have to be expensive or extravagant, simply thought through.

- Suggest an activity in which you (1) have something in common and (2) will get a chance to talk about it at some point; Going dancing? How about a stroll afterward. Movies? Suggest a coffee after to discuss it.

- When you suggest it, suggest it clearly. A vague request is nobody's friend. For some people this can be the most difficult part. Some examples that work better than "Wanna get together sometime?" include:

"I thought you might be interested in [insert name of sporting event/art gallery opening / something interesting] happening [insert specific date and time], would you like to come with me?"

or

"I am super excited about [insert concert/title of movie/cooking class/ whatever]. I'm going [insert specific date and time]—I'd love it if you'd want to come with."

## During a Date

- Remember good hygiene is pretty important to most people.

- Small talk is as well; balance out asking them questions about themselves and taking the emotional risk of sharing info about yourself. Be interested, be honest, be yourself.

- Unless it is the point of the date, like a church picnic or political rally, politics and religion tend to be problematic conversation topics, and there are loads of other subjects you can focus on.

- Meeting "There" is a great way to reduce stress—so is getting there five minutes early.

- In terms of safety, make the first date public, always have enough cash on you to pay your own way, and make sure you have a way to get yourself home on your own.

- Being a queer person, there is no need to avoid any physical displays of affection or attraction to your date, but it's smart to be cautious. "Accelerating Acceptance," a recent study by the Gay and Lesbian Alliance Against Defamation, found that most Americans are becoming more accepting of public, LGBT displays of affection but there is still an approximate third of the population (29 percent actually) that report being somewhere between "somewhat" and "very" uncomfortable seeing a queer couple holding hands.[1] *So*, there's that—making it still important to pay attention to your level of PDA, and doing it consciously and with awareness of your surroundings and potential audience while doing so.

- If you can (and especially if you did the asking), offer to take up the check, but don't let it devolve into a wrestling match.

- It's always cool to split (if they buy the tickets—you get the popcorn, they buy dinner / you get drinks, they paid the cover for the concert / you spring for dessert and coffee after).

## Speaking of After

- Unless they were an absolute creepshow, no one ever died from giving a date a hug and a thank-you.

- If you don't want a kiss, substitute a handshake for the hug.

- Be open to the kiss. Create an opportunity (but do not force) a quiet moment with some eye contact—if it's a go, you will know.

- If they shook your hand—it's not gonna be a go.

- If you don't think you will call or text them for a second date, then do not say you will.

- If you did have a good time (or said you would call or text), then call or text within two days, max.

- If anything happens below the clothes or below the belt, call the next day.

If you identify as trans (or outside the typical gender binary), one extra layer of dating involves **the Ifs, Whens, and Hows to tell your partners about your gender identity.**

## The First Is the If

Your safety should always be your primary concern. Many people you date are going to respond with acceptance, but not everyone. Some potential dates (especially males) may feel threatened or respond with negativity and even violence.

## The Second Is the When

Some people feel more comfortable getting to know someone and letting someone get to know them before coming out with the more personal details of their gender identity.

Others think it is easier on them (and more respectful for the other person) to be upfront about it right away.

## Finally, the How

Public places are a smart option; this helps make sure any negative reactions stay under control. Also smart is to have an exit strategy. Ensuring you have your own way to get out of there and home safely means you will not be stuck in an awkward or dangerous situation (and will avoid the possibility of a freakout on their part in the car).

Other best practices include keeping your phone charged, choosing public places at which you are a regular and recognized, and the not-necessarily-old-fashioned practice of introducing your dates to parents, roommates, friends, or your buddy the barista when they come to pick you up.

---

### LGBTW . . . Online Dating

Online dating is creative, commonplace, exciting, and exhausting. In this day and age, you are officially more likely to ask / be asked out via a screen than in real life.

To be clear, when online (just like in real life), there is a difference between hooking up (getting together for the purpose of sex) and dating. Many hookup apps try to disguise themselves as dating apps, and many people (particularly male-identified people) use dating sites as hookup sites. Be aware of this when using dating apps and sites. It can be hard to find other out, interesting, and interested, attractive and attracted queer people, but this is not a good reason to jump into hookup apps that are designed for adults and can be dangerous for teens.

Online dating is legit, and many people are meeting, creating great relationships, and even getting married through online dating, though it more often results in a couple of dates and a fade-away. Still, there is

---

something magical about spending time becoming clear about what you want (and don't want) in a partner, and then putting that out there for like-minded people to respond.

However, online dating should really be called online meeting. It's a great way to make a connection, but not for actively connecting. It's great for speed and volume, but not always substance or actually getting to know another person. Many people have become trained to automatically choose or reject while screening potential relationship prospects, as though we are scrolling through an Amazon wishlist. Relationships are more than swiping right or hitting the "like" button.

Online dating can put you in contact with interesting people quite easily, but it's important to remember that the work of actual emotional and physical intimacy is harder. Relationships involve things like being vulnerable (as opposed to posting a staged selfie), wanting to be with a specific someone (not amassing an endless queue of online profiles), transparency and truly being seen (not as a curated profile), emotional expression (not an emoji), cuddling (not an upvote), and eventually being naked with someone (as opposed to a sultry photo).

The good news is that online dating can help you build muscles of banter and conversation that can make face-to-face discussions in real life easier as well. Just remember that online dating is meant to create opportunities for real-life intimacy. If real relationships were as easy as the ones online, everyone would be in one.

# RELATIONSHIPS

Dating is only the beginning. Once you begin dating and partnering with people, you will have to be prepared to negotiate and navigate relationships—not just with the people you date, but potentially with friends and family as well.

## Get Comfortable Being Single

Everyone is their own best advocate, but if you are any flavor of queer, then being your own best advocate can be even more important. Take the time to know and understand, and accept and be proud of yourself before you share that self with someone else. In service of "If-You-Can't-Love-Yourself-Why-Should-Anyone-Else?," don't look at being single as a bad thing. People who need others to feel complete or good about themselves sometimes make bad choices in order to be with those others. Being comfortable spending time with just you will help you make good choices around partners *and* make you a better partner for them.

## Be Cool

No one likes to be rejected. If you're not interested, or no longer interested, be nice about it. Also be clear about it. As a therapist and sex educator who has worked with teens for the past several years (and I was once a teen myself), I know how difficult it is when the person they're interested in is not clear. It feels less civilized but is actually much more humane to offer a clear "no," if that is what the answer is. Vague and noncommittal answers are nobody's friend. In general, most people would rather have clarity than a cushioned ego, a definitive answer rather than the prolonged ache and confusion of wondering and hoping.

## Be Cautious

In rare (but still-too-often) cases, turning down a guy (and they are usually cis guys) might lead to aggression—those guys are out there—but the vast majority will not respond to rejection with violence. If you have or get the sense that a rejection may prompt violence, then vague and noncommittal is the way to go.

## Breaking Up Is Hard to Do

Powerful people speak their minds and let the other person do the same. They are honest, nonviolent, and accept responsibility for their choices, instead of trying to place blame on the other person. Breaking up with someone is different than asking someone out (see above regarding bravery and class). If you have seen someone in their underwear, then you must break up in person. Breaking up with someone via text is both cowardly and lame. Choose not to be That Person. Ghosting (deciding you aren't interested anymore and disappearing without an explanation or closure) is not cool. Don't be them, either. When you must break up with someone, do it quickly, not publicly, and nowhere near the date of the other person's birthday or a major holiday.

## Stay Friends with Your Exes

The ability to remain friends with exes, and friends who were "almost," is typically a sign of a good person (as opposed to the person who *can't* be friends with any of their exes or almosts). People notice that stuff.

The general pool of GLBTQ people is much smaller than that of straight/cis people, but one thing that all people have in common is that dating sometimes ends in a breakup.

It is in your best interest to work to end things well and clearly when a dating situation does not work out. Chances are always high that you will see your ex again, and in queer culture, it is also a distinct possibility that you will see your ex on the arms of another out friend (possibly even another ex)—you'll see them at the club, the rallies, the gym, the weddings and parties, play with and against them at the softball games. . . .

Of course nice, neat splits do not always happen and staying cool with each other afterward is not always possible, but it *is* a good goal—with such a relatively small, queer world, it isn't wise to go around burning bridges.

## Mates Before Dates

Or cliques before chicks, buds before studs—whatever you wanna call it, friends are forever. Romantic partners? Not always so. A partner who doesn't want to know the people who are important to you, doesn't really want to know you. See above re: the high likelihood of running into each other in the future and remember not to burn any unnecessary bridges (and be weary of those who do).

## Mind the Gap

Speaking of friends. . . . At some point, you will likely get crushes on your straight friend/coworker/roommate/barista. Statistically there are many more straight people than gay people on the planet, and you will interact with them. Tread carefully. You can't necessarily control your feelings, but you can control your responses to them and your behavior.

One of the suckiest parts of life, which everyone (regardless of gender or orientation) deals with at some point, is the pain of having strong feelings for someone that aren't returned.

Some romantic relationships are just not good ideas, not meant to be, or not even possible, and trying to force the issue can offend, alienate, or hurt the other person.

Would you want someone trying to change your orientation?

It takes time to get over someone, but you can make the process easier (and yourself happier) by getting out, keeping busy, and enjoying time with friends. If you have a particularly close friendship with the person, you might be able to tell them how you feel without making it weird. If you can't talk about it or move on, then taking a break might need to be the answer.

There may also be times when a straight friend comes onto you. They may joke, flirt, or even make a move at some point. Sometimes this can be someone's way of testing out the waters—maybe they think they are not straight and want to see what it's like on the other side, maybe they want to experiment just for fun, or maybe they have an emotional connection to you that they think needs to have a physical component too. Communication is key in this situation, though a conversation about it may make questioning their identity or orientation "too real" for them.

This is also a tread carefully moment. If you want to be that person for them, that is a legitimate choice. Just keep in mind that, likely, this is because they trust you and feel safe with you, so it is very important to be careful with their heart.

It is also important to be careful with your own heart. Regardless of how much they feel safe with you, they still have to deal with the rest of the world and their place in it tomorrow. They may have a hard time dealing with their feelings and/or anything physical that might happen, and they may get weird. If this happens, try not to take it personally—it's not about you, but about what you represent to them. You may represent a life they can't have or a freedom that they can't take. You may represent an unattainable or lost love, a past identity they can't let go of, or a future that is too scary for them to deal with. They may take this out on you, stomp on your heart a bit through the process, and/or no longer be able to be your friend afterward.

Bottom line: being a person that can be trusted in this way is an honor, and a gift you can give someone, but (ironically) it could end up costing you that friendship.

## Mind the Other Gap

The other queer teens and young adults you will meet will be in different stages of their coming out. Acknowledgment (the coming out part) and acceptance (being comfortable about being out) are also different things, and not every teen is going to be at the same stage in their development. So be cool. Don't shame or force labels or yourself on anyone who isn't ready yet. Offer them acceptance for who and where they are; encourage them and ask questions and be patient. It can be tricky to date someone who is not out if you are. They may feel pressure to come out quicker than they are comfortable, though more likely, you will feel pressure to step back into some closets, and that is not the healthiest choice.

## Keep It PG in Front of the Family (Mind the Visuals)

This is good manners for everyone: gay, straight, cis, trans, teen, or grown-up. Your family members don't want to see you making out and groping someone else any more than you want to see them doing that. Of course, you don't have to closet yourself or anything, and you can be loving and affectionate with your partner in front of your family, but nothing that couldn't be shown on the Disney channel.

And, speaking of your parents . . .

## What To Do If Your Parents Hate Your Partner

At some point you will have a partner whom you will want to introduce to your family. This can be a big step in a relationship, but also a big step individually as a statement of integrity.

Sometimes this goes swimmingly, and sometimes, for even the most supportive parents, having the actual evidence that your child is not straight or cis sitting across from you at Thanksgiving can bring up issues.

Work hard to sort any weirdness out as soon as possible; Romeo and Juliet is an amazing play (#Shakespeare!), but no one wants to live it out in real life (spoiler alert: no one wins).

**So, here are ten things you can do:**

### (1) Talk to Your Parents

By asking specifically what it is they don't like, and giving them a chance to verbalize what they are thinking and feeling, you give them an opportunity to either (A) understand that their reservations are based on emotional rather than rational concerns, *or* (B) make a solid point based on legit concern for your best interest (parents do that sometimes). By doing this:

You will be acknowledging that you do care about them, and that you value their opinion and that you appreciate them caring about you.

You can address and investigate reasonable concerns, if they have them.

You can explain and dispel any unreasonable or misguided issues they bring up.

Even if you don't like what they have to say, at least you will have shown them and your partner respect!

### (2) Unplug. Wait 30 Seconds. Restart.

The-Big-Partner-Intro can be a huge step, and it can be easy to forget that it is also The-Big-Parents-Intro. If you have already tried an introduction, but botched it because you made it all about you and your right of passage in unveiling your partner for the very first time, try again and remember to also make it about your parents. Make sure you give your partner some background: a list of things to talk about (and things definitely to *not* talk about), a heads-up about some likes and dislikes (Mom loves hyacinths, Dad hates reality television, Grandma is a teensy bit racist) . . . work to set everyone up to succeed.

### (3) Remember the "One Year" Rule (see chapter 8)

It extends to your significant others as well . . .

### (4) Limit Contact

If it takes longer than needed to sort it out (or you find you just can't or they just won't), try to only have your partner and your parents in the same room at the same time when you absolutely must. When you do, keep it low-stakes, try to stay on neutral ground, and make sure no one feels trapped—make sure anyone can find an elsewhere to be if they need to.

### (5) Increase Contact

Alternatively, trying to find shorter, but more frequent opportunities for them to be in the same room can also help thaw frosty interactions. Meeting out in public for coffee dates, shopping trips, quick stop-bysjust-to-say-hi, or even dinners out in public can help increase familiarity and desensitize stressed out people.

## (6) Find Common Denominators

It may be hard, but working to find *some* crossover in interests between your partner and parents can really pay off in the end. Historical fiction? Buddy cop movies? Thai food? Hating the 49ers? Encouraging them to talk to each other about things they both like or doing things together that they both enjoy can reduce the awkwardness. It's all about showing them that they have more common ground besides you.

## (7) Don't Force It

If they just do not get along, don't force it. The more you push the harder it's going to be, and they may all discover in the end that what they do have in common is resenting you for pushing them. Be sensitive to them as much as is reasonable. You don't need to not take sides—it *is* possible to be on everyone's side.

## (8) Discourage Them from Interacting via Social Media

The distance of screens makes it very easy to say things one wouldn't necessarily say in person. Insist that everyone keep things civil and not do or say anything that cannot be undone or unsaid should they decide at some future point that they can get along.

## (9) Go Zen

You have a partner that cares. You have parents that care. Be happy, grateful, and proud.

## (10) *Really* Limit Contact

Yes there may come a time at which you may need to choose between them. Try not to burn any bridges, but it is your life and they can hate each other if they want to.

Put energy into both relationships, try to find fulfillment from both as well, and do your best to stay out of the middle. Compartmentalizing is a queer superpower—half of you reading this will have had to deal with divorced parents (and half of those will have been through the breakup of a parent's second marriage[1]). Guess what? It's the same muscle group! You got this.

---

## LGBTW . . . Dating Older People

Although teens are exiting the closet at increasingly younger ages, ironically, it can still be difficult for LGBT youth to find each other and participate in some of the romantic rites of passage their straight/cis counterparts do.

Some young queer people gravitate toward older, more experienced queer people. This is not uncommon in the GLBT teen community for several reasons:

- It can be hard to meet openly LGBT people your age.

- Youth, who have been forced to leave home because of their sexual orientation or gender identity, may find other adults that can offer things that their parents can't, like a place to live and financial support.

- You can learn things from an older, more experienced queer person. They can answer questions and guide you as mentors. They're ahead of you on their path and can be excellent guides for you on yours.

- Straight people get to start making those sweet dating and romantic mistakes in middle school. Many queer people find themselves not having the opportunity to do this until their late teens or early twenties, and having an older advocate can help.

Sometimes having relationships with people older than you can involve (or evolve) into dating people older than you, but it's very important to understand the challenges and dangers that can come along with dating someone significantly older.

**Does your relationship feel equal?** Equality is one of the theme songs of queer folk. If you have an older partner who is controlling, or makes all of the decisions, doesn't value your opinions or your wants, "parents" you

---

(like making you ask permission to do things / go places or being in charge of all the finances), then your partner is not interacting with you like an equal. If you feel like you're being controlled, you probably are.

**Dating older people can be culturally difficult.** Yes, they have more stories and life experience to share, but if you're dating a partner who has never heard a Beyonce song, who remembers when MTV played music videos, still says things like "land line," is proud of the fact that they don't text, or looks forward to *not* having plans on a Friday night, it can cause friction and/or boredom in the relationship.

**Grown-up and growing up are different things.** Don't miss out on your teens, and early twenties. Though being queer in your teens can be a very different experience than being cis or straight, that experience builds character. It contributes to that life experience that you might find intriguing in an older person, and helps you to become who you are meant to be. When we fast-forward through our teens or early twenties, by dating someone older, and jumping directly into an adult lifestyle, you risk missing out on some really important, valuable, and formative experiences. Plus suddenly being "grown up" without actually growing up can be very stressful. Yes, things like prom and spring break can be kind of lame, but so can mortgages and dinner parties.

**There are laws. Serious laws.** The age of consent in many places is somewhere between sixteen and eighteen, and those lines are drawn for good reasons. Yes, there are benefits to being exposed to older, wiser people, but there are just as many benefits to building relationships with people who are in the same developmental stage as you.

The differences between someone who is twenty-six and someone who is thirty-six are much, much smaller than the differences between someone who is twenty-six and someone who is sixteen.

The thirty-six-year-old is going to be more established in their job/career, have likely had more relationships, may have a different relationship to technology, or a larger savings account and a different coming out process, but generally they will be dealing with the same things in their day-to-day life as the twenty-six-year-old.

The sixteen-year-old's life and the twenty-six-year-old's life should look very, very different.

Statutory rape refers to sex between someone who is over the age of consent (which is typically between sixteen and eighteen) and someone who is under the age of consent.

When this happens—even if it is "consensual," the older person can be charged with a sex crime, and even made to register as a sex offender. Ageofconsent.com is a good resource to familiarize yourself with the age laws in your area. Respecting these laws is a good idea.

There are many positive, healthy, well-meaning, and well put-together older role models in the world that hopefully you will have the good fortune to come across.

There are also manipulative, lecherous creeps out there whom you will also come across, and it is important to keep your radar tuned for them—because they will have their radar tuned for you. A young, possibly naïve, potentially emotionally or financially needy queer kid is like a wet dream to those people.

When you encounter an older person who is giving you a noticeable amount of attention, energy, or gifts, keep your head (and your pants) up until you get to know them.

Some things to keep in mind:

- Does this person have a history of only dating significantly younger people? That could be a sign of a problem—choosing to not date people your age is different than not being able to. You may be mature for your age, but are they *immature* for theirs? Are they dating *you* or are they into teenagers? If you are one in a longer list of younger partners, ask some questions.

- Most adults are exceptionally aware of the age laws I just mentioned (they are the ones who get in trouble, right?), so if you are interacting with an older person, and they begin to try to turn the relationship sexual, be *very* cautious—that is a sign that they are (A) not aware of the riskiness of their behavior and/or (B) do not care.

- In addition to doing what is best for them, an older person in your life should also have your best interests in mind. So an older partner who is encouraging you to use substances, have sex without safety measures, who isolates you from supportive people or encourages any kind of illegal behavior, does *not* have your back.

Be smart and safe when contemplating sex with older people. There are differences between teens and adults (both emotional and legal) that need to be considered.

It is a good idea to seek out opportunities to get advice from trusted, older, and wiser GLBT friends or family members who have been there / done that and can speak to their own experiences. If you are still in high school, it is safe and smart to keep your dating and romantic partners within an age range of about two years.

It can be tough to find other out, queer, young adults, but it's definitely not impossible. You can work to find other gay teens locally through your GSA/QSA or an LGBT youth center in your area, or you can use the Internet and apps to make connections with LGBT teens both near and far.

## LGBTW . . . Trans-Fetishism

Some people's interest and attraction and attention to trans people can be negative.

Of course, it is natural to be curious about what it means to be a trans person or even to feel safe around the confidence and freedom that trans people can exude, but there may be times when it is specifically a person's "transness" or their trans vibe that someone is attracted to, rather than the trans *person* themselves. This is called trans-fetishism, and it's generally not considered very cool.

Being open and interested in dating trans people definitely is cool, and probably a sign of a good person.

However, there are some people who are attracted to trans people at the exclusion of cis people.

The equivalent would be being attracted to a cis woman (or man) *just* because they are a cis woman (or man). There's a difference between being open to dating Asian people or blondes or heavy people and *only* dating Asian people or blondes or heavy people.

These people view trans people differently than "real/normal" people. They focus on one thing (rather than the person), and leave the impression that if a magic wand was waved, and the person were de-transed or suddenly made cis, then their attraction would wane, like the blonde who goes brown or the heavy guy who loses weight.

# CHAPTER FIFTEEN

Some trans people don't have a problem with people who seek out trans partners, but others feel that it delegitimizes them, unfairly reducing people to just one, biological aspect of themselves that doesn't represent their whole identity or experience.

# INTIMATE VIOLENCE

Healthy relationships all look different. For queer relationships, there can be even more variation—including how they're structured, who's in them, and how those who's identify themselves. The world can be harder, more stressful, and even more actively hostile for queer people than it is for straight/cis people. Your relationships should be safe spaces for you to be as much you as you can be.

There are many things that factor into a relationship, including

respect
honesty
trust
fairness
talking/listening
boundaries
support
love
sex

Some signs of a healthy relationship include:

- Respect for each other's chosen gender pronouns and name.

- Respect for each other's boundaries.

- Never threatening to out each other to others.

- Never telling each other you're not a "real" lesbian, gay man, trans person . . .

- Not teasing each other about how you define, do, or desire sex.

- Not forcing each other into doing/not doing certain sexual acts.

Some relationships are healthy, some are unhealthy, and some healthy ones have unhealthy parts that need to be paid attention to.

**Good partners:**

- **Do not try to control you.** Preventing you from having friends, interfering with your choices, or giving you orders are signs that your partner is controlling. You do not have to put up with this.

- **Do not emotionally abuse you.** Some people need to tear you down to make themselves feel better (or at least make you afraid to leave them because they seem like the only one who would ever put up with the mess that is you). This is called emotional abuse, and you don't have to put up with this, either.

- **Do not disrespect you.** Good partners are not afraid of equality. A partner who is condescending, insulting you or putting you down about your thoughts, feelings, brain, body, or heart is not a good partner. A partner who is constantly explaining how they are more powerful/smart/interesting/whatever than you are is only trying to convince you that you are "less-than."

- **Do not invade your privacy.** In a healthy relationship, there is no need to hide big things from your partner. That being said, privacy is a thing. Your partners don't need to have your passwords, access to your feeds, or the right to snoop through your bags, journals, or tech. Doing so without reason or consent is creepy, and should not be tolerated.

- **Do not use trust as a weapon.** Having someone distrust you when you've done something untrustworthy is legitimate. You know yourself; you look at yourself in the mirror before you go to sleep at night. If you legitimately have done nothing to earn someone's suspicion, then don't put up with it. Do not start a game of trying to earn trust from someone who mistrusts you for no reason. That is a game that can't be won.

- **Do not make you feel too far down their list.** A relationship is a part of life, not life itself. Just as no partner should ever be a higher priority on your list than you are, your partner should be focused on his or her own goals, self-worth, and individuality. You should not expect to be number one on anyone's list but your own. Number two is a great position to shoot for, but there are times when things like school, jobs, physical health, parents, or (eventually) kids may need to take a higher slot on our own lists. These things shift and morph as time passes and intimacy grows. However, if you find that you are consistently lower down on your partner's list than you want to be, talk about it. Being a priority is different than being a primary focus or an afterthought.

- **Do not make you do all the work.** A relationship is about teamwork. Relationships can become difficult as energy levels, personal feelings, and emotions fluctuate. The ups and downs of the rest of our lives invade our relationships. We need to be prepared for this to happen, ride the waves, and do our legit best for our partners. And we should expect them to do this, too.

- **Do not avoid conflict.** No one particularly likes conflict, but problems can't be resolved until they are faced. Avoidance of difficult topics and situations stops a relationship from progressing and potentially makes the problems worse.

- **Do not cheat on you.** There are plenty of examples of monogamy not being the natural, default state for humans. Some people may not be wired to spend long periods of time with one person. But if you are clear about your commitment and expectations, then a good partner is going to do her or his best to hold to that commitment, and take responsibility and repair it if they don't.[1]

## LGBTW . . . Dating Violence

Dating violence (also called intimate, partner, or relationship violence) is abusive, aggressive, and controlling behavior in a relationship, either straight or gay. People who are not in a romantic or a dating relationship can do intimate violence to each other as well.

**There are different types of intimate violence.**[2] **The most obvious are**

- **Physical abuse**, like hitting, kicking, choking, or anything that leaves a bruise, and

- **Sexual abuse.** This includes things like rape, non-consensual touch, and limiting access to safer sex techniques, but also includes anything that takes away your ability to control how, where, or when you engage in sexual contact.

**Intimate violence also includes**

- **Verbal (also called emotional) abuse** like insulting or threatening you, isolating you from friends or family, and stalking, and

- **Digital abuse**—using the Internet and other technologies to harass someone else. Things like sending unwanted messages, non-consensual images, invading privacy, cyberbullying, threats, and cyberstalking.

LGBT youth can be perpetrators of violence as well as victims.

According to a 2013 report from the CDC,[3] about 10 percent of high school students reported experiencing physical or sexual dating violence, with lesbians and gay men experiencing equal or higher levels of intimate partner violence as heterosexuals.

A 2016 study released by the Centers for Disease Control and Prevention[4] showed significantly higher rates of dating violence among LGB youth than among non-LGB youth; 17.5 percent (compared to the 8.3 percent reported by straight youth) for physical violence and 22.7 percent (compared to 9.1 percent) for sexual victimization within relationships. Transgender youth report the highest rates of dating violence, with a shocking 88.9 percent reporting dating violence.

Abusive people do not tend to stop without some sort of consequence, classes, or counseling—in fact they tend to get worse. Dating violence is particularly confusing, because it involves someone you care about and who supposedly cares about you, and (again) the bulk of stories you tend to hear about in media involve straight, married couples, so there can be a myth that this doesn't happen in queer relationships or to teenagers or it doesn't count if you're not married. But it does. One out of every three teens is a victim of dating violence,[5] and hitting anyone—particularly a boyfriend or a girlfriend—is a crime.

**If you have a partner who puts their hands on you (but not in a good way)[6]:**

- **Leave**. It is not your fault. Do not make excuses for them. Continuing to be in a relationship with them communicated to them that their behavior is OK, and will mess with your ability to separate appropriate behavior from appropriate behavior.

- **Block**. Unfriend, unfollow, change any passwords you shared with them (or that they found out), set your profiles to private and block them from texting or calling you. Full dark/no stars: if you respond after their thirteenth message, then you have only succeeded in telling them the next time they will only have to message you fourteen times . . .

- **Tell**. Talk to other people to get support.

The best thing you can do is to be watchful for signs of abuse, both against yourself and others, and say something if and when you see it.

**Signs of an abusive relationship[7] include a partner who**

- checks your devices, social media accounts, or email without permission;

- uses actions to show anger (rather than words);

- shows jealousy (with anger);

- shows insecurity (with anger);

- is constantly putting you down;

- isolates you from family or friends;

- makes false accusations;

- physically hurts you (in any way);

- tells you what to do; and/or

- pressures or forces you to have sex.

If you or someone you know has been a victim of dating violence:

- Tell your parents, a teacher, or another concerned adult.

- Call the National Teen Dating Abuse Helpline: (866) 331-9474 (or text "loveis" to 22522).

- Call your local police.

---

## LGBTW . . . Don't Be "That Person"

Being young, being new to relationships, and/or coming from an abusive background are risk factors for being That Person. Having testosterone in your system, any kind of attention deficit issue, or poor emotional management (like anger or depression) up the chance of you abusing a partner as well. Stress, poor social skills, and substance abuse don't help either—but talking to someone about those things will.

**If you are or (have been/might be) abusive toward a partner:**

- Talk to your family, your doctor, or school counselor.

- Call a local intimate violence resource in your area, and ask for a referral to a therapist.

- Call the National Teen Dating Abuse Helpline: (866) 331-9474 (or text "loveis" to 22522).

## PART FIVE
# "SOMEWHERE OVER THE RAINBOW"

Individual sexual tastes can be as compatible or incompatible as our tastes in music and food. What one person likes, dislikes, wants, or needs, another may find scary, gross, or intimidating. Many people spend a good deal of time developing their sexual tastes in isolation or entering into relationships for the first time having given very little thought to what turns them on (or off). Either way, merging our tastes with someone else's can be both awkward and fun.

## CHAPTER SEVENTEEN
# THE SEX PART

The Internet and other media we consume can be full of stereo-typed myths and biased misinformation that lesbians should be aggressive but other women should be passive, that all gay guys like anal sex and men should have 10-inch penises, and that everyone else should enjoy it when they do.

We are taught that sex goes on for forty-five minutes and involves a dozen position changes, that everyone always knows what they are doing, they orgasm every time they have sex, and of course do it at the same time as their partner. (Again: most do not.)

There are no universal positions or patterns that work for everyone.

- It's important to be clear for yourself where your lines and definitions are.

- It's important to be sure that you and your partners are on the same page about your definitions.

- It's important to ask about different types of sex when talking to partners about their sexual histories.

- It's important not to assume what someone's definition or activities are based on how they identify.

- It's important to use protection and safety measures no matter what kind of sex you have.

**Orgasm** is when muscular contractions of the penis (for natal males) or vagina (for natal females) and anus (both) create intense feelings called an orgasm. For many people, this is often accompanied by ejaculation.

**Ejaculation** is the discharge of the fluid (also called "come" or "cum"); orgasm is the big, good feeling. Orgasm and ejaculation are *not* the same thing. Though they often happen at the same time, they are different processes.

Both male and female bodies ejaculate. Bio males ejaculate about a teaspoon of semen, containing approximately six hundred million spermatozoa.[1] There are so many of them because sperm are very sensitive and easily damaged by time, temperature, the inhospitable environments of mouths and anuses, and the acidity of both the urethra and the vagina. During conception, for example, fewer than one thousand sperm will make the journey all the way to the egg, and (usually) only one gets in.

The female body's counterpart to the prostate, technically known as Skene's glands, is embedded in the wall of the urethra. Just like the prostate, the ducts from these glands create secretions (similar to semen but without sperm) that lubricate the vagina, and some people can actually expel (or ejaculate) this liquid from their urethra.

Both male and female bodies orgasm. Although the experiences are similar, there are differences between the male and the female orgasm. Biological men reach orgasm most typically through the rubbing of the head of their penis (the glans), but can also reach orgasm through stimulation of their prostate. Bio women reach orgasm through vaginal penetration (with fingers, penises, or tools and toys such as vibrators or dildos, in order to stimulate the G-spot), but almost 80 percent of people with vaginas also need clitoral stimulation to achieve orgasm.[2] Many people masturbate by only rubbing their clitoris.

Orgasms from stimulation of the glans or clitoris tend to focus inward (picture the Death Star's laser at the beginning of *Star Wars: A New Hope*). Orgasms through stimulating the G-spot or prostate tend to focus outward (think of the Death Star blowing up at the end of *Star Wars: A New Hope*).[3]

---

## LGBTW . . . Wet Dreams

Some people experience orgasms while sleeping. These are called nocturnal emissions or, much more commonly, "wet dreams." These can happen while dreaming about sex, though not necessarily. They may wake you up, though not necessarily, and may leave evidence in the form of a discharge (that's

---

the "wet" part), particularly for people with penises. Not everyone has wet dreams, though everyone can. Having male hormones in your system may cause you to experience them more frequently. Most people have fewer and fewer as they begin masturbating, become sexually active, and grow older.

Orgasm does not need to be the be-all-and-end-all, whole point of sex. Orgasm does not mean that everything went right and everyone got what they wanted. Not having an orgasm does not mean that something went wrong. There are plenty of things to do and plenty of fun to be had without that big finish. Keep in mind that your largest sexual organ is your skin, and your most important sexual organ is your brain.

**Masturbation**, also known as "jacking off," "jilling off," and a bunch of other hilarious euphemisms, is achieving orgasm by stimulating your own genitals. Masturbation can also be done by other types of bodily contact, with objects, or to other people.

Most people who have a clitoris masturbate by rubbing their clitoris with a finger. Some use lubrication; others prefer a dry hand. Some people with vaginas rub up against pillows or vibrating devices. Some enjoy penetrating their vagina with a finger or dildo (see below). Some masturbate while lying in bed, sitting in a chair, or lying in the tub (though strive to not leave the water running for long periods of time; the earth is in terrible shape).

People with penises typically masturbate by rubbing their penis either with an open palm or a closed fist. Some prefer lubrication; others prefer a dry hand. Some also rub their penis against pillows, or inside intricately balled-up tube socks. Some enjoy penetrating their anus with a finger or dildo. People can masturbate while sitting, catching their semen in the palm of their hand. People can let it land on their stomach while lying on their back in bed or wash it down the drain while masturbating in the shower.

Because of centuries of religious teaching and some vague idea that some people share that masturbation can be harmful, masturbation in some cultures has been associated with shame, guilt, and anxiety. Some people have received negative messages about masturbation from their family or religious leaders, but the reality is that masturbation is a natural expression of sexuality that has many benefits. Masturbation reduces stress, muscular tension, and can help you sleep.[4] It also allows you to become more familiar and comfortable with your own body and internal sex life and can be a way to express sexual feelings with someone else, while avoiding the risks of disease or pregnancy.

Masturbation can be done with or to other people, though it is typically a solo activity. Your bedroom or bathroom is likely to offer you the most privacy—masturbating in other places such as the living room, kitchen, or someone else's bedroom are usually frowned upon. In fact jilling or jacking off in public places, such as school, in a car, or anywhere near a webcam, can be illegal depending on where you live and how old you are.

---

## LGBTW . . . Sex Toys

Sex toys are devices designed for penetration of the vagina or anus, and are used by people of all genders and orientations for masturbation (and sometimes during sex with a partner).

There are lots of different kinds of sexual toys, ranging from quite small to quite large and from silly looking to a bit scary. The two most common types are vibrators and dildos.

Vibrators are cylindrical wands that contain batteries and can be switched on to (you guessed it) vibrate pleasurably.

Dildos are similar in shape to vibrators, but don't typically vibrate. They can be made from wood, glass, metal, plastic, or rubber, and are often shaped to look like an actual penis (or some kind of mutant, summer blockbuster action movie version of one).

Vibrators can be rubbed on a clitoris, penis, or around an anus. Some people insert them into their vagina or butt. Dildos specifically designed for anuses are typically called butt plugs. They have a flared base on one end to prevent them from being completely inserted and/or lost in (and later embarrassingly removed by emergency room staff from) someone's butt.

Sex toys such as vibrators and dildos can help you develop a relationship with your own body, provide a safe way to be sexual without involving another person, and be a nice way to safely explore sexual feelings (with or without a partner).

Sex toys are generally difficult for minors to purchase, but through the Internet all things are possible. The reputable online retailers smittenkittenonline.com and babeland.com also specialize in answering questions in nonjudgmental ways.

---

It is possible to physically harm yourself by masturbating too hard, too much, or by masturbating in an unsafe manner. The number one rule is to stop if you cause yourself pain. Other important rules on the list include things such as:

- making sure anything going into your vagina or butt will come out.

- nothing breakable or that could cut or burn (see above re: pain).

- avoiding toys with any cracks, rust, or plasticky, new car smells.

- keeping your toys, hands, and fingernails clean.

- remembering to use lube when needed and necessary.

- using barriers such as condoms and lube (especially with anuses).

- reserving toys for personal use—no loaning, borrowing, or leaving them out for company to find.

Not everyone masturbates or masturbates regularly, although most people do—it's estimated that approximately 90 percent of women and almost 95 percent of men masturbate.[5] Masturbation often begins in adolescence and continues through adulthood. Although most people do it, masturbation is still not a common topic of conversation for most people.

**Sexual fantasies** are like daydreams of things that excite us and turn us on. Like other kinds of fantasies, these thoughts can be ways to explore and rehearse things we may hope to try in the future, just like we have thoughts of fame, fortune, or the future. Like other kinds of imaginative thought (such as superpowers or living through a zombie apocalypse), sexual fantasies may involve things that are unrealistic or that we would never actually want to do in real life.

Most people pair sexual fantasy with masturbation, but it is also typical to sometimes think sexual thoughts while doing other things like falling asleep or sitting in class. In fantasy you can imagine yourself in different locations doing different activities with different people—some you may know, celebrities you may never meet, or people you create in your own head.

Just like masturbation helps us explore and learn more about our own body, fantasies can help us get clear about our internal sex life—we can try on different aspects of our personality or orientation. We can learn many things about ourselves by paying attention to our sexual fantasies, which can help us better communicate our desires (and limits) to future partners. Some people find fun in sharing their fantasies with other people, even if they are choosing not to do the things they are talking about until later.

Having a fantasy life is both healthy and safe. However, if you find yourself fantasizing about things that are disturbing to you, find yourself thinking about things that would be unethical or illegal in real life, such as rape, or sex with animals or children, or feeling plagued with constant fantasies that feel hard to turn off—a qualified therapist can help.

Bottom line: There is nothing wrong with you if you masturbate. In fact, the only times masturbation can be harmful is when it becomes compulsive: when it takes up so much of your thoughts, time, and energy that it starts to cause problems in other areas of your life.

This is also an argument against pornography, as the two things are unfortunately linked on a fairly regular basis. Obsessive or compulsive masturbation and/or use of pornography (like all other behaviors that someone has difficulty stopping) are signs of an emotional problem that needs to be addressed with the help of a counselor or therapist.

---

### LGBTW . . . Pornography

Every second, 28,258 Internet users in the United States are viewing pornography, according to Top Ten Reviews online. There are sixty-eight million search engine requests for porn each day—that's 25 percent of all online search requests![6]

People are being exposed to pornography online at younger and younger ages, often by accident, while playing games, surfing YouTube, or doing homework.

Pornography is designed to sexually excite people; this is a typical marketing ploy that works very well. Porn does not turn people into perverts or monsters, but it can have an impact on the ways in which we look at (and operate in) the world. Viewing pornography on a regular basis can have harmful and damaging effects, especially during adolescence when we are forming our ideas of who we are and what we are aroused by.

**Porn**

- is a (very poor) substitute for sexual education,

- portrays unrealistic ideas of sexual interaction,

- can distract from actual relationships,

- can lead to negative imprinting to and arousal by unhealthy or illegal things,

- can weaken or atrophy one's own imagination and capacity for fantasy,

- can out you if discovered, potentially putting you at risk for violence,

- can be expensive,

- can be habit-forming.

Choosing to incorporate pornography into an existing sexual lifestyle as an adult is *very* different than constructing a sexual lifestyle built on pornography. Chances are that some of your sexual partners will have used pornography as their primary source of sexual education. Particularly if you date male-identified people, you may encounter some partners who think they know how to "do sex" because they have watched so much porn. However, although the things you see in online pornography are *sexual*, they are not necessarily actual *sex*.

If you do choose to look at porn:

- make sure you jack/jill off using only your imagination at least half the time.

- work to not let it impact how you treat other people.

- do not let it impact how you feel about yourself.

If you are trans—whether you feel confident about your gender identity or are just figuring things out—you may not always feel completely comfortable in your body, which can make sexual behavior complicated.

Perhaps you do not feel comfortable having other people touch your genitals or other specific parts of your body, or maybe there are specific sexual acts you don't want to do.

That is OK.

There are plenty of ways to feel connected.

There are plenty of ways to feel sexual pleasure.

**Kissing** is one of the few sexualized acts that involves all five senses; sight, sound, smell, touch, and taste. Because of this kissing can be incredibly intimate, even though it is often one of the first things people do when they are attracted to each other.

The basic components of the modern, romantic kiss are eye contact, a hard-to-describe / kinda magical "moment" with a slight gravitational pull followed by a tilt of the head so your noses don't hit. Most people kiss with eyes closed and twice as many people tilt to the right rather than the left.[7]

Putting your tongue into the other person's mouth (or letting them put theirs into yours) is commonly called "French" kissing. This does not mean wagging your tongue around like a dog out a window or trying to suck someone's ribs up through their neck. Most people learn through trial and error, but it never hurts to ask for feedback.

Hickeys are bruises caused when one person sucks someone else's blood to the surface of their skin. The bruises can last anywhere from a couple of days to a couple of weeks. Some people are OK with hickeys, though many others see them as a very "middle school" thing. Having a hickey on your body could be embarrassing, could make you look immature or irresponsible in the eyes of others, and could get you in trouble at home or work. Hickeys should never, ever be done to someone without consent or on a place they can't cover up.

**Oral sex** is when one person puts their mouth or tongue on the genitals of another.[8]

The scientific name for oral sex on a penis is fellatio, but typically it is called a "blow job"—even though there is no actual blowing involved.

The scientific name for oral sex on a vagina is cunnilingus, but typically it is referred to as "eating someone out"—even though there is no actual biting involved.

Guidelines for performing oral sex on a penis[9]:

- No teeth!

- Don't be afraid to use your hands.

- Think ice cream cone, not banana.

- Deep-throating (when someone takes someone else's entire penis into their mouth and throat) is a porn thing. It is varsity-level stuff, and takes specialized training and/or practice. It rarely ends well in real life. A lapful of whatever someone had for lunch earlier is not sexy. Do not try.

- Don't forget the testicles. Jiggle (don't squeeze) them, tug (don't pull) them, and stroke them (like the top of a cat's tail, not the back of a dog's ear).

Guidelines for performing oral sex on a vagina[10]:

- Do not go straight for the clitoris.

- Tongues hurt unless they are lubricated.

- Do not wag your tongue about like a dog out a window.

- Spelling the alphabet with your tongue (or their name . . . or the lyrics to your favorite song) is fun for everyone.

- Use your fingers, as long as your nails are short and clean.

- Keep your nails short and clean.

For everyone:

- Ask for feedback.

- Give feedback.

- Reciprocate. *Do not* ask anyone to put their mouth anywhere that you are not willing to put yours.

- Condoms and dams are a good idea to use every time!

**Vaginal sex** (when penis-vagina) involves one person moving their erect penis in and out of another person's lubricated vagina. This can be done in several positions, though the most common is referred to as the missionary position—the one you see straight/cis actors performing in movies, lying face-to-face, with the person with the penis on top and the one with the vagina lying underneath them.

Still reading? Yes, the missionary position may not be anything you may be interested in or planning on doing, but since it is so popular in mainstream media (and typically the only one talked about in most mainstream sexual education classes), it is important to remember that, despite what those movies lead us to believe, it is not the only kind of sex. In fact it is not even the only position in which people do vaginal sex. Partners can be facing each other, "spooning" (with one person's back to the other), sitting or lying down—the options are not endless, but there are more than the missionary position, though all of them involve the penis going into the vagina.

**Anal sex** (when penis-anus) involves one person putting their penis into the anus of another person. And it *does* count as sex. P.S., so does oral sex. Even though some people leave that part off when they talk about

---

## LGBTW . . . Saddlebacking

Some people actively choose to engage in oral sex and/or anal sex, but still consider themselves virgins. Typically this is done for religious reasons, and some vague, shaming value around the concept of purity. Though the concept and definition of virginity can be complicated and customized, when someone is creating or maintaining such a disconnect between their values and behavior, they are not going at sex like a grown-up.

---

it, saying, "We did anal last weekend," or "I got oral last night," it still counts, and should be treated with the same level of respect and safety as penis-in-vagina sex.

During anal sex, in general, the person doing the penetrating is referred to as the "Top," and the person being penetrated is called the "Bottom." Neither is any better than the other (well, depending on whom you ask), but they are descriptors that make talking about anal sex easier.

With hetero couples, the definitions and defaults of "doing it" are more limited. If two straight kids want to, plan to, or have sex, it almost always ends up with a penis in a vagina. When two queer people are engaged in sex, that term can mean many different things, and so queer folk tend to (out of necessity) engage in more detailed discussions about what they may or may not end up doing at the end of the night, and terms like "top" and "bottom" help.

*And*, anal sex is not a just a gay thing. Statistically, only 50 to 80 percent of gay males engage in anal sex.[11] According to the National Survey of Family Growth, it is a regular feature in approximately one-third of heterosexual couples.[12] Anal sex is generally more pleasurable for people with prostates than it is for people without prostates, but there are many nerve receptors in the anus, and anal play can feel good to lots of people.

Just like with oral sex, reciprocation is important. Anyone who wants to stick anything up your butt should be willing to have the same thing done to them. This creates empathy, and encourages them to be as gentle and safe with you and your parts as they want you to be with them and theirs.[13]

All sex acts should be as safe and pleasurable as possible for both people involved. Regardless of what kind of sex you may be having—ask questions along the way, and always listen to what your partner says.

## LGBTW . . . Again, Pornography

Porn is sexual, but it is not *sex*. Porn is fantasy; it is not real. Those people are actors, and the entire thing is scripted. Not only does porn tend to show unrealistic bodies doing unrealistic things, but (like any other fiction on film) they don't tend to show all the outtakes and things that take place in between scene changes, like showers and coffee breaks.

- Despite what you see in porn, anal intercourse is not something to be done spontaneously; it is a slow, patient process.

- Despite what you see in porn, stretching is a big part of the prep. Start with fingers first.

- Despite what you see in porn, lube is important to help avoid both the pain and trauma that can result from improperly attempted anal sex. (#AnalFissure)

- Despite what you see in porn, do not go from anus to mouth (or vagina for that matter). Intestinal parasites are a concern and hepatitis is an even bigger one.

- Despite what you see in porn, the bottom (the one being penetrated) is the one in charge.

- Despite what you see in porn, never let anyone put a penis in your butt without a condom on.

- Despite what you see in porn, dental dams should be used when putting a mouth on someone's anus (also called analingus or more commonly, "rimming").

- Despite what you see in porn, pain is not sexy—it is nature telling you that you need to stop.

Vaginas produce their own natural lubricating fluids. The amount and effectiveness of each person's **lubrication** varies throughout their lifetime, and their monthly cycle, but the fluid they produce makes penetration easier.

Anuses are *not* self-lubricating, and anal sex without the addition of a lubricant can be very painful, and can increase the risk of condom breakage and damage to the thin lining of the rectum, allowing HIV virus to enter the body.[14] The risk of contracting HIV as well as other STIs is higher for anal sex than any other kind of sex. In fact, according to the CDC, the probability of the receptive partner catching HIV during unprotected oral sex with an HIV carrier is one per ten thousand acts. During anal sex, it's fifty per ten thousand acts. This means that anal sex is fifty times more dangerous than oral sex.[15]

Some lubes are specifically designed for anal sex; look for water-based lubes with just a touch of silicone.

There are four main types of lubrication: glycerin, silicone, natural oils, and petroleum-based.[16]

**Glycerin lubes** are water-based, which means that they can be washed off with water, and when they dry out, they can be reconstituted with water as well. Glycerin dries fast and absorbs into the skin, so these lubes need to be reapplied or reconstituted often. The sugars in glycerin can contribute to yeast infections in women and should not be used if you are diabetic or if your immune system is compromised. Glycerin does not stain sheets or eat away at condoms, but glycerin is an ingredient in laxatives, so do not use it for anal sex, because . . . yeah.

**Silicone lubes** are a less sticky and longer-lasting form of water-based lube, because the silicone prevents the lube from drying out. Most lubricated condoms are made with silicone. Not all silicone lubes are condom safe, although most are; check for a label that says "CE." Silicone cleans up with soap and water.

**Natural oils** are typically plant- or vegetable-based and safe to eat, which means they are safe to put inside your body; however, *they will destroy condoms*. These are best saved for massages and masturbation.

**Petroleum-based lubes** are oil-based, synthetic (artificial), and not digestible. They can also cause irritation inside vaginas and anuses, destroy condoms (making the spread of disease easier), and they don't have any antibacterial properties. These lubes include things like Vaseline, lotions, or hair conditioners. Don't use these for sex.

## CHAPTER EIGHTEEN
# ABSTINENCE AND INDULGENCE

Abstinence means not doing something—generally it means not engaging in sex with other people. People who are abstinent find other ways of giving and receiving sexual pleasure besides penetration.

Some people limit their sexual play to kissing, hugging, or fondling. Some feel OK doing more than that, some less. The choice to be abstinent can be made for many reasons and can be a long-term decision or a short-term one. Everyone has to decide when and if they are going to engage in sexual activity. Though most people become sexually active eventually, some never do. Some wait to engage in active sex with another person until they are in a significant or long-term relationship. Some wait for marriage, some college, some prom night, some this weekend. . . .

Everyone is only abstinent until they decide not to be.

People who are abstinent sometimes make the mistake of not educating themselves to be prepared for when they do decide to engage in sexual contact, because it doesn't feel necessary. But like knowing how to swim, drive a stick shift, or perform CPR—even if you're not doing it right now, it is still important to prepare yourself for later . . . just in case.

Anyone practicing abstinence should also be educated and have a backup plan.

The decision whether or not to remain abstinent should not be something that one has to feel ashamed of. Do not let someone intimidate, guilt, force, or otherwise manipulate you into making any decision about your own body. What you do with your genitals is no one's choice but your own.

Just like no one should force, coerce, or manipulate you into having sex, no one should be making you choose to *not* have sex, either. Indulgence is the opposite of abstinence, though—just like abstinence, it is a choice. When and if you choose either, make sure you are doing it for your own reasons and not someone else's. Part of growing up is learning what (and who, and when) is right for you.

**Virginity** is a super-vague term that generally refers to someone "who hasn't had sex." The vagueness lies in the fact that the word *sex* can be a very relative term—meaning different things to different people. This can be especially true if you are not straight. If two straight people want to, plan to, or have "sex," they are almost always going to be referring to someone's penis eventually ending up in someone's vagina. For queer people, that is not necessarily the default. Queer people have both the necessity and the opportunity to speak more specifically about the acts that they are interested (or not interested) in doing. Because of this (more so than their straight counterparts), queer people's definition of what "sex" means, and therefore what "virginity" is, is more complicated.

Sex between GLBT people (and the conversation around it) is different than it is for straight people. There is a lot about straight sex that is assumed (mostly that at some point a penis is going to be aimed at a vagina), but in queer relationships, sex can mean different things. A great conversation starter is "What are you into?" or "What turns you on?" This encourages your partners to tell you what they like and don't like and paves the way for you to do the same.

If you are willing to be naked with someone, you should be able to discuss the names of specific body parts and sexual acts, safer sex methods, and what your limits and boundaries are about all of that. If you can't talk about these things, you shouldn't be doing them.

As a relationship becomes more intimate, communication should expand to include sexual behaviors you have done in the past, fantasies about things you want to experience in the future, and bigger picture concepts such as orientation, gender, and what virginity means to you.

The first few times you talk about these things may feel awkward, but with practice, it gets a little better each time as you and your partner become more secure in yourselves and your relationship.

The more times that you have these conversations, the more comfortable you will both become. In the meantime, if it is more difficult to have a conversation with your partner about sex than it is to actually *have* the sex, that's a good indication that you might want to wait a bit longer.

Virginity, in reality, is like a candle, not a lightbulb.[1] It diminishes with time and experience. It is not turned off or on like a switch. It is also not something one "gives" to or "takes" from another person. There is no "V card." It's a whole deck, with dozens of little virginities along the way. There is the traditional and literal "virginity"—meaning you've never had sexual intercourse. But there are dozens of other physical and emotional types of virginity, too, like your first crush, first kiss, first naked time with another human, and first exchange of bodily fluids.

Overemphasizing one specific act at one specific time can lead people to do things that they do not like or that are not right for them. Every new experience and partner can be important, even game-changing, and can bring feelings (both physical and emotional) that you have not felt before.

There is no clear rule about when someone is ready to have sex with someone else. Ideally, you are ready for sex with someone else when your mind, heart, and crotch are all balanced and working in sync.

But keep in mind:

- Crotches are usually ready before hearts.

- Hearts tend to come online before minds.

- Minds can be taken down relatively easily by hearts and crotches (as well as pot, booze, porn, not enough sleep, too much caffeine, certain songs, other people's crotches, shiny stuff . . . ).

For most people, the mind, heart, and crotch don't sync up until at least age sixteen, and for many people not until twenty-five.

# CASUAL SEX

Casual sex typically refers to one of two kinds of sexual relationships: friends with benefits and hookups.[1]

**Friends with benefits (FWB)** relationships are sexual, but not romantic, relationships between otherwise platonic friends.

Reasons people enter these kinds of relationships include

- to explore sex or sexuality with someone they trust,

- to experiment or "learn the ropes" in a safe context,

- just for fun.

More negative reasons people enter these kinds of relationships include

- hoping they can eventually turn it into a romantic relationship.

- mistakenly thinking that their body is the most interesting currency they have to exchange in a relationship or get attention.

- wanting to get the physical benefits of a dating relationship without any intention of following through on the emotional responsibilities.

FWBs are tricky for a couple of reasons. Sometimes, people get emotional (once the sex starts) in ways they did not anticipate, and get weirded-out or uncomfortable trying to stay casual after doing such intimate things with someone. Other times, when/if one of the partners becomes sexual with someone else besides their with-benefits friend, there can be issues of loyalty, jealousy, trust, and personal safety (such as the increased risk for STIs).

The keys to a successful, FWB situation are safety, communication, and balance.

- Do it for reasons that work for everyone.

- Follow the same safer sex guidelines that you would in an actual dating relationship.

- Check in regularly to make sure that both people are OK with the nonromantic relationship.

- And remember that the most important letter in FWB is the F—not the B.

A successful FWB relationship requires varsity-level maturity, decision-making, and communication skills, and should not be taken lightly, despite its perceived casualness. Until you are an actual adult, the most responsible way to view an FWB situation is as legit practice for future dating relationships—not as an alternative to them.

**Hookups** are different than FWB relationships. Hookups (or one-night stands) are generally considered sexual interactions that happen spontaneously between people who just met or do not know each other well. Hookups can involve anything from making out to actual penetrative intercourse, and may or may not be the beginning of an ongoing relationship (though, typically, it is assumed that they are not).

Hookups are things. They are not necessarily unhealthy—but/and when you are considering sexual contact without the anchor of relationship, the chances of someone being harmed both emotionally or physically can increase the more casual your casual sex is.

# PART SIX
# "CLOSER TO FINE"

Practicing responsible, preventative sexuality can include getting yourself tested regularly, making good choices (like not having sex while under the influence of substances), and being able and willing to have uncomfortable and honest conversations with your partner/s. But, prevention specifically means protecting yourself from disease and/or pregnancy *every time*.

## CHAPTER TWENTY
# SEXUALLY TRANSMITTED INFECTIONS (STIS)

Currently, there are more than a dozen separate organisms and syndromes classified as sexually transmitted infections.[1] Infections that are spread through sexual activity have been known by several names over the centuries, including social diseases, venereal diseases ("VD"), and "STDs" (for sexually transmitted diseases). Though, currently, these are referred to as sexually transmitted infections or STIs.

The reason for this is that the word *disease* implies an obvious medical problem, complete with signs and symptoms. But many STIs are caused by bacteria or viruses that do not have clear signs, or have symptoms that can go unnoticed for long periods of time, so the term "infection" is more accurate.

**The ten, big, bad STIs are grouped into the following three categories**:

> **bacterial**: gonorrhea, chlamydia, syphilis, and pelvic inflammatory disease
> **parasitic**: crabs (lice and scabies) and trichomoniasis
> **viral**: herpes, hepatitis B, HPV, and HIV/AIDS[2]

That last group—the four H's—are by far the scariest. This class of STI is systemic and includes viral infections that affect organ systems other than just the reproductive system. There are no known cures for these viruses, although there are vaccines to prevent against two of them (below).

## The Bacterial STIs

**Gonorrhea** is a microscopic bacterium that spreads via vaginal, anal, and oral intercourse. Gonorrhea causes sterility, arthritis, and heart problems, and a pus-like discharge from the urethra, which causes pain during urination.

Condoms and dental dams offer very good protection against gonorrhea, but both partners can be successfully treated with oral antibiotics. Often, people with gonorrhea also have chlamydia and must be treated for both infections at the same time.

**Chlamydia** is a sneaky bacterium that has few symptoms in the beginning, but will cause painful and burning discharges during urination and intercourse, inflammation of the rectum and cervix, swelling of the testicles, bleeding after sex, and, eventually, sterility. It is spread through vaginal and anal intercourse, and there have been cases of passing the parasite from the hand to the eye.

Chlamydia is easily prevented with condoms/dams and (if caught early enough) treated with antibiotics for a week. Chlamydia can be misdiagnosed and confused with gonorrhea. In fact, most women and half of the men who have this disease do not know that they have it, and are still spreading the disease. Three million American men and women become infected every year.[3]

**Syphilis** is a sexually transmitted organism (called a spirochete) that causes three phases that go in no particular order, often overlapping and causing different, distinctive symptoms. One phase starts with painless, crater-like sores around your genitals or around your mouth, which ooze a highly infectious liquid. Without antibiotics, a month later, a painful rash appears on your palms and the soles of your feet.

Another phase lasts for years and has no symptoms, which is highly unfortunate because, if left untreated, syphilis progresses to the final phase, which involves hair loss, brain damage, physical disfigurement, paralysis, and death.

Condom use and antibiotics are your best and only defense against syphilis. Damage done during the late stages cannot be undone.

---

## LGBTW . . . The Bacterial STIs

As of this writing, chlamydia, syphilis, and gonorrhea have risen for the first time in more than a decade, according to the CDC.[4] The highest number of infections is among people in the fifteen- to twenty-four-year-old range,

---

including two-thirds of all reported cases of chlamydia and gonorrhea.[5] It's likely that if you are reading this book, you fall within that age range.

Because chlamydia and gonorrhea (and one of syphilis's phases) often have no symptoms, many of these bacterial infections go undiagnosed, making it even more dangerous for young people who contract them, and making it easier to spread it to others.

Chlamydia, specifically, has climbed to 1.4 million annual cases in the United States.[6] This is the highest number of annual cases of any condition ever reported by the CDC. Ever. As in: The history of everything, ever.

This is preventable with condoms. As a species, humans have achieved massive breakthroughs in technology and advancement, such as the Internet, artificial hearts, GPS, the Human Genome Project, and Tivo. There is zero reason this should be happening right now.

Due to a host of factors, including the total failure of abstinence-only education, bacterial STIs are likely to continue to (literally) plague the population born after 1990, so the responsibility to stop them falls on your shoulders.

If you're smart enough to read this book and clever enough to download apps that connect you to other humans, then you can find some condoms or dental dams and figure out how to use them (see chapter 22).

The best ways to avoid contracting and spreading these infections:

- Limit your number of sexual partners.

- Use condoms/dams consistently and correctly. Use a barrier. Every. Single. Time. (Yes, even during blow jobs. That's a thing now—get into it.)

- Set up a regular testing schedule for yourself. Once per year is the minimum requirement to be able to consider yourself a responsible sexually active person. Choose a day for your yearly STI screening, say, August 14 (exactly six months after Valentine's Day, a nice cap to any summer adventures and a fresh start to the school year!). Put it in your calendar app.

- Go ahead, I'll wait.

- Seriously, do it now.

- No, you won't remember later.

Back? Thank you. Now, let's add in **a little formula**:

For every additional partner you are sexual with throughout the year, cut your time between testing in half. So, two partners per year would mean testing every six months. A third partner would mean getting yourself tested every three months, and so on.

It is also important to remember to ask your clinic to test for all of the major STIs when you get screened. Some clinics do not automatically screen for herpes or HIV, for example, unless you specifically ask.

**Pelvic inflammatory disease (PID)** is a serious infection that develops when an infection spreads from the vagina and cervix into the reproductive organs. PID is usually the result of a sexually transmitted infection such as chlamydia or gonorrhea. Those infections are spread by vaginal and anal intercourse and, sometimes, oral sex. Insertion and removal of IUDs can increase one's risk for PID as well. If PID is not treated, it can cause serious problems, such as infertility, ectopic pregnancy, and chronic pain.

Condoms offer very good protection against PID. A health care provider can diagnose PID during a pelvic exam. Tests will also be done for chlamydia, gonorrhea, or other infections, because they often cause PID. PID is treated most often with antibiotics and a period of bed rest and abstinence.

## The Parasitic STIs

**Crabs** are also called "pubic lice," "scabies," and "cooties." This is an easily transferred STI that not even barriers can prevent—because these infections are caused by actual bugs. These tiny, gray bugs attach to your skin, turn darker when swollen with blood, and attach eggs to your pubic hair. They resemble tiny crabs, live off of your blood supply, and make you itch like a crazy person.

Treatment consists of a couple of doses of special lice shampoo. The dead crabs (and their eggs) have to be pulled out of your pubes with a tiny comb. Wash clothes, bed sheets, and so forth, with hot, hot, hot water and some of the shampoo. The only protection against this infection is to limit your number of intimate and sexual contacts, and avoid people who don't. Other things that can help prevent this include washing clothes from used-clothing stores before wearing them, steering clear of people who can't stop scratching their crotches, and avoiding sleeping in sheets that do not seem clean—especially if they are on beds of people you don't know very well.

**Trichomoniasis** is caused by the single-celled protozoan parasite, *Trichomonas vaginalis*. The vagina is the most common site of infection, although the urethra in men can also be affected.

Most guys with "trich" do not have signs or symptoms, but some feel irritation inside the penis, discharge with a strong odor, or a slight burning after urination and ejaculation. Symptoms usually appear within one to three weeks of exposure, but the parasite is harder to detect in men than in women.

When someone has been infected, both partners should be treated at the same time to eliminate the parasite. People should avoid sex until both partners finish treatment and have no symptoms. Latex male condoms, when used consistently and correctly, can reduce the risk of transmission.

## The Viral STIs

**Herpes** is a virus that takes two forms: simplex 1 and simplex 2. The first one is associated with cold sores or fever blisters. The second type involves hot, itchy blisters that burst open and create ulcers.

Both can be transmitted sexually and start out with flu-like symptoms, followed by a recurring rash, which includes clusters of the tingly sores (simplex 1 on the mouth; simplex 2 "down there," "back there," "under there," and everywhere in between). Once infected, symptoms can be triggered by stress and include painful burning during urination.

Herpes is most contagious from the time when sores appear until the scabs fall off, but some people can be contagious even when they do not have symptoms. Mucous membranes of the mouth, anus, vagina, penis, and the eyes are especially susceptible to infection. One million new cases are diagnosed every year.[7]

Dental dams and condoms help to prevent herpes, but only when the sores are not already present. Medications can decrease the number and intensity of outbreaks, but herpes is not curable, and like many other viruses, remains with you for life. Don't touch anybody anywhere with any part of you that has sores until they heal; wash your hands often; and do not touch the sores.

**Hepatitis B (HVB)** is a virus that is transmitted sexually and through all bodily fluids. It is very sneaky and very, very, very contagious. In the beginning, it causes extreme fatigue, headache, fever, and vomiting. Later on, symptoms include yellow skin, brown urine, and attacks on the liver, which lead to cirrhosis, cancer, and possibly death. Almost forty thousand Americans get HVB every year (and an estimated 1.2 million people in the United States have it right now).[8] Hepatitis C (HVC) can be spread by sex as well, but much more rarely, and is more associated with drug and alcohol use.

Barriers offer some protection against HVB and HVC during vaginal, anal, and oral intercourse, but the virus can be passed through kissing and other intimate touching. In some cases, the infection clears up in a couple of months, but some people remain contagious for the rest of their lives. HVB is preventable with a vaccine, but only if you get it before exposure. If you were born before 1991 and/or did not get it as an infant, go and get it. Now. Hepatitis is more than 100 percent more contagious than HIV.[9]

**HPV (genital warts)** are cell-mutating human papillomaviruses that come in approximately ninety different varieties and cause a variety of itchy, flesh-colored, cauliflower-like warts. This disease is spread through genital contact, with or without symptoms. There are a few strains of HPV that do not manifest as warts, but that's not good news; these varieties can cause cancers in the cervix, vulva, and penis.

Genital warts can be prevented with dams and condoms, and can be treated with suppression medications, professional freezing, topical creams, lasers, and acids in places you really don't want lasers and acids. A vaccine has been developed (go ask your doctor!), but at this time, there is no cure. Rumor has it that after several years you can "grow out of it," but this has not been proven.

**HIV (human immunodeficiency virus)** is a viral infection that can weaken the body's ability to fight disease and cause acquired immune deficiency syndrome (AIDS)—the last stage of HIV infection. HIV is spread through blood, semen, and vaginal fluids. HIV remains in the body for life and is the most dangerous of all STIs, causing weight loss; constant, uncomfortable diarrhea; purplish growths on the skin; pneumonia; a variety of cancers; and death.

HIV is prevented through condom use and can be managed with drugs. It is incurable, currently fatal, and at this time, no one has recovered (see chapter 21).

## LGBTW . . . Vaccines

Two of the most serious STIs now have vaccines available that can help prevent you from becoming infected. The first vaccine is for hepatitis B. Depending on which of two different vaccine types your medical provider carries, a series of two or three shots over a six-month period is given to people between the ages of eleven and eighteen. It has been part of the recommended immunization schedule for babies born after 1991 in the United States.[10]

It is important to find out if you have received the vaccines because, although HVB is generally considered an adult disease, it is extremely contagious, and underagers can get infected as well. Thanks to the immunization, HVB infections have dropped 95 percent since routine immunization began in the early 1990s,[11] although the CDC estimates that approximately one million people in America carry HVB in their blood, and five thousand people a year die from this virus.[12]

There is also now a vaccine that prevents the types of genital human papillomavirus (HPV) that cause most cases of cervical cancer and genital warts. The vaccine, Gardasil, is given in three shots over six months. The vaccine is routinely recommended for people ages nine to twenty-six, especially if they are sexually active.[13]

It is theoretically possible that, if every young person with a cervix can be vaccinated once they become sexually active, cervical cancer may be eliminated completely in future generations. But do not be fooled by the assumption that HPV is a "girl" thing because the vaccine is pushed for natal girls and associated with cervical cancer. A 2011 study from the H. Lee Moffitt Cancer Center and Research Institute reported that half of all male-identified Americans might be infected with the human papillomavirus.[14] The HPV vaccines are approved for natal males ages nine to twenty-six as well, and along with condoms, are two of their biggest weapons against HPV.

Our third weapon against HPV is our immune system, which clears most HPV infections with little difficulty. However, the strain HPV-16 is connected to mouth, throat, head, neck, and anal cancers. HPV can be spread through oral and anal sex, as well as vaginal sex.

If and when you choose to become sexually active, it's almost guaranteed that you will be exposed to some strain of the nearly one hundred different types of HPV (genital warts being one of them). Vaccinating can benefit everyone by preventing genital warts and rare cancers, such as penile, cervical, and anal cancer.

Important facts about STIs:

- More than eighteen million Americans contract an STI each year.[15]

- Nine million of those people are between the ages of fifteen and twenty-five.[16]

- There are ten thousand new diagnoses every day. This averages out to one every eight seconds.[17]

- The CDC estimates that half of all young adults in the United States will contract a sexually transmitted infection by age twenty-five.[18]

If you think, or worry, or know that you have been exposed to any STI, follow these three steps:

- Don't panic.

- Don't ignore it. Get checked out and treated by a doctor as soon as possible. Taking a friend, partner, or supportive adult with you is also a good idea. A visit to a doctor will provide you with helpful info, a decrease in your stress level, probably a bit of tough love, and some medication, if you need it.

- Don't have sex again until you're done with any prescribed treatment.

Sexually transmitted infections happen. There is no 100 percent safe sex, just as there are no 100 percent safe salad bars or 100 percent safe drivers.

Do your best to use safety measures, though if you do get an infection (and many of you reading this will), do not let it affect your self-esteem. Contracting an infection does not make you a bad person any more than food poisoning or fender benders do (which many of you reading this will also experience).

# HIV/AIDS 101

The human immunodeficiency virus (HIV) can infect and live in your body while slowly weakening your immune system, which is your body's mechanism for fighting off infections.[1]

Specifically, HIV attacks a type of white blood cell called the T lymphocyte (or T cell). T cells help defend against infections and diseases. If HIV enters the body, it attacks a T cell and slowly works its way inside the cell. Once inside, the virus takes over and uses the cell as a virus-making factory to copy itself. The newly made viruses then leave the T cell and go on to infect and destroy other T cells. This is how HIV multiplies. Once a T cell has been invaded, it can no longer fight illnesses within the body.

The T cell range in the typical human is between 500 and 1,800 (typically 800 to 1,200). When a person's T cell count drops below 200, their immune system is considered compromised (too weak to keep them safe from infections). This is called acquired immune deficiency syndrome (AIDS).

AIDS makes us very susceptible to other bacterial and viral infections that we would normally be able to fend off. AIDS doesn't kill you—it makes you die from other things. Even things such as the common cold, which is easily fought off by healthy immune systems, can become very dangerous.

Being infected with HIV and having AIDS are two different things.

Someone who is infected with HIV is called HIV-positive. Being HIV-positive does not necessarily mean that someone will progress to full-blown AIDS. Some people can stay relatively healthy and free of symptoms for several years or even longer with medications that are available today. The term "poz" has been embraced, particularly in the gay community, for people who are HIV-positive.

People are diagnosed with AIDS when they have a very low number of active T cells left and show signs of a serious infection. There are thirty-three AIDS-defining illnesses, called opportunistic infections, which take advantage of weakened immune systems.

Twenty years ago, having AIDS meant that you were dying. Today, the situation is different, thanks to medication regimes that can slow down the virus's progress. However, even though researchers understand the virus more and more each year, AIDS is still considered fatal.

HIV is spread through blood, semen, vaginal secretions, and breast milk, but blood transmission is most common. Transmission occurs when any of these four infected fluids move from one person's body into another's through

- unprotected sex with an infected partner

- sharing needles during drug use

- transmission of fluids from mothers to babies during childbirth or breastfeeding.

People who have another sexually transmitted infection, such as syphilis, genital herpes, chlamydia, or gonorrhea are at greater risk for getting HIV during sex if they have an infected partner. Some STIs increase risk because of the presence of sores, but any infection in the body will trigger the immune system to attack with more T cells, which the HIV virus feeds on.

Although an HIV-positive person may look and feel healthy, the virus is silently reproducing itself and destroying more and more T cells. It can take a while for someone's body to recognize that it is under attack or to show symptoms, which is a major factor in why the disease is still spreading. In fact, every month, one thousand young Americans become infected with HIV.[2]

People have been fighting HIV since the 1980s, when most children infected with HIV were born with it. We have learned so much, and developed so many protections and interventions that it is simply unacceptable that young people in this country are being infected in such high rates.

It is possible to find HIV in the saliva, tears, sweat, and urine of infected individuals, but there are no recorded cases of infection by these secretions. Animals and insects do not pass on the disease, nor can HIV be transmitted by sharing silverware, water, food, toilet seats, or even hot tubs and swimming pools with infected people.

The CDC reports that latex (or polyurethane) condoms are highly effective in reducing the risk of HIV transmission.[3] The risk is lower for the penetrative partner than the receptive partner (in general). Oral sex has a relatively low risk because of the low pH levels in the mouth and enzymes in saliva that kill HIV. Any anal sex causes microscopic tearing and invisible amounts of blood, which increases the risk of HIV. There are also studies that have shown that HIV can penetrate healthy, intact vaginal lining.

Just as overactive immune systems increase risk of HIV infection, so do compromised systems, so eating right, exercising, getting enough sleep, and stress management are important risk-reduction tools as well.

Just because someone is exposed does not mean that they will be infected. Testing is important and best done within three months. Between 90 and 95 percent of infected people will have enough antibodies to show up in a test within the first twenty-five to thirty days after infection; by the three-month mark, almost everyone who is infected will test positive. After that three-month mark, HIV rapid tests can be taken at public health clinics, and results can be obtained in as short a time as twenty minutes.

There are two tests. The first is the enzyme-linked immunosorbent assay (ELISA) test, which screens for antibodies. A negative ELISA test means you are HIV-negative. A positive ELISA test means you need to take a second test, a western blot test, which screens for the virus itself. A person needs a positive response on at least one of these tests to be diagnosed HIV-positive.

After exposure to HIV, there is post-exposure prophylaxis (PEP), which is a month-long medication regimen that greatly decreases the likelihood of infection, especially if taken within twenty-four to seventy-two hours of infection. The medications are usually available in emergency rooms, and work by stopping the infection before it reaches the lymph nodes. The meds are extremely hard on the body and quite expensive, ranging from eight hundred to two thousand dollars for a month's supply.

Pre-exposure prophylaxis (**PrEP**) is an anti-HIV medication that keeps HIV-negative people from becoming infected. It is most commonly referred to by its prescription name, **Truvada**. Truvada can be used in two different ways.[4] Though it can be used in people as young as twelve who have already been exposed to HIV to treat their infection and manage symptoms, it can also be used (along with other safer sex practices, such as condoms) to reduce the risk of being infected with HIV by someone else. Unfortunately, right now it is only approved as a preventive measure for adults (eighteen and older).[5]

Truvada is a daily pill that has been approved as safe and effective by the FDA. It stops the HIV virus from being able to duplicate itself, interfering with its ability to create an infection. Truvada does not cure HIV or AIDS, but when used properly it has been shown to reduce the risk of HIV infection by as much as 92 percent.[6]

PrEP is a smart option for anyone who is at greater-than-usual risk for contracting HIV. This includes

- anyone who is in an ongoing relationship with an HIV-positive partner;

- anyone who is (or dates) a gay or bisexual man who has had anal sex without a condom or been diagnosed with an STD in the past six months;

- anyone gay or straight (or other) who does not regularly use condoms during sex with partners of unknown HIV status (and who are at substantial risk of HIV infection, e.g., people who inject drugs or have bisexual male partners);

- intravenous drug users.

If you are older than eighteen and fall into one of the categories listed above, PrEP may reduce your risk of contracting HIV.[7] Your doctor can give you a prescription or direct you to a medication assistance program.

Whether or not you fall into any of the categories above, always practice safer sex techniques (such as choosing less risky behaviors, consistent testing, communication, and condom use), and never share needles with anyone for any reason.

# LGBTW . . . Poz Shaming

**Poz** is the "nickname" for HIV-positive gay and bisexual men. Like slut-shaming (bullying or humiliating someone who has sex), poz shaming often holds a tone that lots and lots of sex led to the infection or diagnosis.

The ironic thing is that a lot of that poz shaming comes from other men who have sex with men, but who are HIV-negative.

The mentality seems to come mostly from the fact that, in a post-1980s AIDS Crisis world, with so many ways to avoid contracting the HIV virus, some dudes just don't have a lot of sympathy or empathy for those who do get it.

The big picture is twofold because incidence of HIV is rising. In fact, young people (aged thirteen to twenty-four) accounted for over 20 percent of new HIV infections in America in 2011. It is thought that almost half of young people living with HIV are not aware of their infection.[8] The "It won't happen to me" attitude is the biggest contributor to this—discouraging young people from testing for HIV. So . . .

One: HIV is definitely still a thing, and behaving as if it is not is simply stupid (and thinking that only certain kinds of people get HIV is stupider on top of that).

Two: This is exactly why we use safer sex techniques that protect against the HIV virus *every time*, right? Including condoms and PrEP. We should enter any new sexual relationship understanding that anyone can have HIV and anyone (including us) can contract it.

Poz shaming shows up most obviously on dating/hookup apps, where the term "clean" (as in, "I'm clean"/"Clean guys only") is tossed about to indicate that someone is disease-free, as if having an STI makes you somehow "dirty."

It can be scary or even intimidating when you meet your first friend/date/sexual partner who has contracted HIV, though it's important to balance that apprehension with empathy, education, and good judgment.

Buffy the Vampire Slayer once said, "There but for the grace of getting bit, go I."[9] *Anyone* can get HIV in various ways, so leaving your judgy-pants at home is always a good idea. People who don't get tested regularly, don't consistently use protection, or who just assume their current HIV status is negative look silly and hypocritical when they throw terms like "clean" around.

It is important to be smart if you're going to be sexually active, and understanding terms like "undetectable" and "viral load" is a big part of gay/bi culture. Responsible people talk to their doctors about ways to remain safe and get tested regularly.

When someone discloses an HIV-positive diagnosis, *thank them* (there's a percentage of poz folks out there that do not do this), then ask some clarifying questions. If you do find that someone contracted HIV because of irresponsible behavior, like sharing needles or randomly engaging in risky, unprotected sex or not using post-exposure prophylactics after being diagnosed, then use your best judgment and know that choosing not to be sexual with that particular person may be a good idea. This is especially important if they try to talk you into unprotected sex.

---

## LGBTW . . . If You Get an STI (Part I)

The infections I've described above can be gross, upsetting, and/or downright terrifying. Sexually transmitted infections at their best are uncomfortable, and at their worst can be life-threatening.

If you think you've been exposed to an STI, or if you are having symptoms that make you worry that you've got one, you owe it to yourself and your partners to see a doctor immediately. There is nothing to be gained by waiting (except possibly a worse diagnosis and more infected teens). If you are old enough to have sex, you are old enough to behave responsibly and face the risks of sex head on. Contracting an STI doesn't make you a bad person, but knowingly or carelessly spreading one does. Get yourself checked out, and get yourself healthy.

Help and support about STIs are available twenty-four hours a day, seven days a week from Planned Parenthood, (800) 230-PLAN (7526), **PlannedParenthood.org**.

Some people let the ickiness of STIs keep them from getting help, but most STIs are treatable or at least manageable. Do not let embarrassment or shame keep you from getting checked or treated.

---

# SAFER SEX

All sexually active people can benefit from proper and consistent uses of contraceptives and/or safer-sex practices. Some of these techniques focus on preventing the spread of disease (safer sex), most deal with avoiding pregnancy (contraception), and some do a bit of both.

---

## LGBTW . . . Reproduction

Only a percentage of you reading this may have sex with someone in which pregnancy is a possibility, but it is still important to be educated on the contraceptive techniques, because people change their minds, experiment on occasion, learn more facets about their orientation, and/or can be convinced, pressured, or forced into having penile-vaginal intercourse.

If you are a natal female (even if you're taking hormones) and you have sex with a natal male (even if they are taking hormones), you can still become pregnant!

---

## Parenthood and How to Avoid It

Being gay or trans does not mean you can't have your own child some day. Adoption (making someone else's biological child part of your family) and surrogacy (making a biological child through medical fertilization with someone of the opposite sex) are always options, but even for trans people who choose medical transition, natal males can bank sperm, and natal females can have their eggs frozen for later use, making biological children at least a future possibility.

The most detailed information about safer sex / contraceptive methods can be found at PlannedParenthood.org and Scarletteen.org. The methods most applicable to lesbian, gay, bisexual, and trans people can be grouped into four categories: natural, barrier, hormonal, and medical.

**The natural methods** use few, if any, additional devices and rely mostly on cooperation and timing, and include **masturbation** (sexually pleasing oneself or someone else using manual techniques and/or instrumental manipulation) and **abstinence**—choosing not to participate in sexual behavior with other people. Abstaining from sex is hard to do for some people, and tends to end at some point for most—anyone practicing abstinence should be educated in other methods and have a backup plan.

**The barrier methods** prevent disease by limiting skin contact and prevent pregnancy by blocking the passage of sperm. These include **dental dams** (ultrathin, often scented latex sheets placed over the vulva or anus during oral sex), **outercourse** (sex with clothes on and sex that avoids penetration of any kind—also called "dry sex" or "dry humping"), male condoms, and female condoms.

**Male condoms** are latex coverings placed on the penis to prevent sperm from entering the vagina, anus, or mouth.

**Best practices for condoms care and use:**

**Use them every time.**
This means every time. Gay or straight. Front or back. Night or day. Because sperm can be present in pre-cum—that clear fluid that sometimes comes out of the tip of a penis when it is hard—and because pregnancy is not the only thing condoms protect against.

**Wear the condom that fits your penis, not your ego.**
Do not be tempted by sizes; wearing a condom that is too big is almost as dangerous as not wearing one at all.

**Be nice to them.**
Use only water-based or silicone lubricant—nothing with oil of any kind in it. Do not use more than one at a time—no doubling up. Store them in your bag, nightstand, or bathroom, not in cars, wallets, or pockets, where they can be damaged.

**Avoid condoms with spermicide.**

Unfortunately, nonoxynol-9 is the most popular spermicide in the United States. It kills both sperm and HIV (yay!), but it also causes irritation to the vaginal and anal walls (boo!), making it easier for HIV to be transmitted through abrasions. Because of this, many HIV, AIDS, and health organizations—including the CDC and the World Health Organization—have called for the sale of condoms that contain nonoxynol-9 to be discontinued.[1] Nonoxynol-9 should never be used for anal sex.

**Load up.**

The more available condoms are, the more likely they will be used. Share with your friends!

**Your body is a gift, wrap it well.**

Be sure to roll them the right way. And if you start rolling the wrong way, toss that condom and get a fresh one (see above re: pre-cum). Pinch the tip to create a pocket. Foreskin should be pulled back before the condom is put on. No doubling up, no recycling, no reusing. And, P.S., they have expiration dates for a reason.

**Take care taking them off.**

Hold the condom at the base when withdrawing. Remove the condom after you pull out and before you go soft. Tie off the condom before throwing it away—no flushing and no leaving it on the floor.

---

### LGBTW . . . Condom Resistance Techniques[2]

According to a study at the University of Washington,[3] people with penises sometimes have the tendency to try to convince a partner to not use a condom at some point in their sexual history.

This behavior is not OK.

Not using condoms puts the receptive partner at risk for pregnancy and/or disease. Remember that someone who doesn't want to use condoms with you has likely also not used them with someone else, upping your chances even more of being exposed to something you don't want.

---

Also, it is about respect.

**The most common tactics people use to avoid wearing a condom are:**

Prospective Partner: *"I'm clean / I just got tested."*

There are loads of STIs that can be asymptomatic (which means someone doesn't know they have it unless properly and specifically tested). Plus, pregnancy is still a concern if a person who is producing sperm is having vaginal sex with someone who is producing eggs.

You: *"Hi, 'Clean / Just Got Tested.' It's not pronounced 'Clean,' it's 'Negative.'*
*I am too, and plan to stay that way. Here's a condom."*
Prospective Partner: *"You're so hot / I'm so horny. Let's just do it."*

A percentage of people have attention deficit issues, but sex is not something to be making spontaneous decisions about. Expect that some of the people you partner up with are going to be hyper-focused, distracted, unprepared, or just don't seem to have enough blood to run both ends of their body at the same time. Carry your own condoms.

You: *"You're right. I am hot. So hurry up and put this condom on."*
Prospective Partner: *"It feels better without a condom."*

Condoms theoretically can cut down on some of the sensitivity for some penises. But if the difference between wearing a condom and not wearing a condom were so great, people would clearly notice a sudden change during the 1.5–3.5 percent of the time that condoms break[4] (and most people do not notice).

You: *"Does wearing a condom feel better than your hand?"*
Prospective Partner: *"I just don't wanna."*

This is the lazy person's approach. At best, they are irresponsible. At worst, they're putting you on the spot in the hope you'll let them get their way. This stance indicates that they are childish and childlike around safety. Do they "not wanna" wear seat belts either? Sunscreen? Definitely do *not* put your own safety in the hands of That Person.

> You: *"Well, I do. Take it or leave it."*
> Prospective Partner: *"What, you don't trust me?"*

Jackass alert! Do not fall for this. This is purely and simply manipulation. Taking someone's insistence to use a condom as a personal insult is an immature, douchey move. That choice is about you taking care of yourself, and has nothing to with them.

> You: *"I'm a safety person. This is my rule for myself,*
> *it's not about you. Is that a problem?"*

Bottom line: Be clear about your policy on protection, be open with your partner about it, and stick to your guns—no exceptions. And That Person—you know, the one who asks *again* after you've already said no? That Person gets to go home and have sex with themselves.

While having sex with people with penises, remember to check occasionally that the condom is still on. Do this by reaching down and feeling for the condom's ring around the base of their penis.

**Here's what to do if a condom comes off or breaks during sex:**

- Do not panic.

- Inform your partner immediately.

- Find access to emergency contraception within the first seventy-two hours (if you or your partner is able to get pregnant).

- Get tested.

Here's what to do if someone takes off a condom during sex without telling you:

- Do not panic.

- Find access to emergency contraception within the first seventy-two hours (if you or your partner is able to get pregnant).

- Get tested.

- Do not continue to date or trust That Person.

- Purposeful removal of a condom without the other person's consent is called "stealthing," and can fall under the definition of rape. You also have the option (and encouragement of this writer) to call the police.

**Female condoms** are a longer, wider form of male condoms, inserted into the vagina or rectum, and held in place with bendable rings at both ends. They are not called female condoms because they are "for girls"; they are called female condoms because they go on the inside. They can be a bit noisy, but if either of you are allergic to latex, female condoms can be worth it.

**The hormonal methods** stop ovulation and prevent the possibility of fertilization. There are various ways for natal females to protect themselves against unwanted pregnancy including **birth control pills**, a slow-releasing hormonal **patch** (brand name, Ortho Evra), a bendable, 2-inch plastic **ring** worn around the cervix for three weeks each month (brand name, NuvaRing) and two types of **injection**—one monthly (brand name, Lunelle) and one every three months (brand name, Depo-Provera).

---

### LGBTW . . . LARC

Long-acting, reversible contraception (or LARC) includes contraceptive **implants** (brand name, Implanon) and intrauterine devices—small, plastic, T-shaped objects inserted into a person's uterus. They contain either copper (also known as an intrauterine device or **IUD**) or hormones (also known as intrauterine system, **IUS**, or by the brand name, Mirena), both of which help prevent the fertilization and implantation of eggs.

If choosing a contraceptive method, LARC should be considered safe and appropriate. LARC methods (with failure rates of less than 1 percent per year for perfect and typical use[5]) are highly effective, and have the highest rates of satisfaction and lowest risk of pregnancy of all reversible contraception.[6]

---

---

### LGBTW . . . Emergency Contraception

Emergency contraceptive pills (or ECPs) are also called "Plan B." These are two increased doses of the hormones found in birth control pills taken twelve hours apart. ECPs are different than abortions in that they do not end a pregnancy, but prevent one from starting if taken within seventy-two hours of intercourse to thicken mucus and prevent the release of eggs.

ECPs, like most abortions, are used by some as a backup when other means of contraception have failed—for example, when a condom tears during penile-vaginal sex. It is also a first line of treatment when natal females are sexually assaulted.

Having a healthy, working relationship with your body—not being afraid of it, and being willing and able to ask questions when something seems amiss—is an important part of prevention. These things become especially important if you are worried that you have been exposed to an STI, or may be or may have gotten someone pregnant.

---

**The medical methods** require the assistance of medical means or professionals and include **sterilization**—severing the tubes that carry sperm (vasectomy), or in which the sperm and egg meet (tubal ligation), and **abortion** (ending a pregnancy via chemicals or surgery). Although many abortions are used as birth control, abortion is by no means a contraceptive and should not be considered as such.

## Pregnancy

If you think you might be pregnant, remember to keep breathing. They are called pregnancy *scares* for a reason.

If it has been less than three days, emergency contraception can reduce the risk of pregnancy.[7] The chances of it working successfully drop with every day that passes, but emergency contraceptive pills can be obtained from your doctor, many pharmacies, emergency rooms, and health clinics. Depending on your age and location, a prescription may be needed. Even after emergency contraception is taken, a pregnancy test should still be done.

Reliable, name-brand pregnancy tests can be found in your doctor's office, in clinics such as Planned Parenthood, and most any drugstore. If you are in a position to be taking a pregnancy test at home, buy two at the store (in case you mess up the first one), pay attention to the instructions and the expiration dates, and it might help to have someone with you.

If you have a negative pregnancy test ("not pregnant"), but it has been less than three weeks since the risk event or you have definitely missed a period, another test should be taken (do not reuse a test). Also, you should make an appointment with your doctor or local health clinic within the next week.

If you have a positive pregnancy test ("pregnant"), you should schedule a visit to your doctor to verify the results as soon as possible. And breathe.

If you find out after testing that you are pregnant, you may be tempted to judge or shame yourself. That energy would be better used finding support and information about options including abortion, adoption, and parenthood.

If you think you might be or find out you are pregnant:

Tell at least one supportive adult in your life.

## LGBTW . . . If You Get an STI (Part II)

Practicing safer sex, including getting checked for STIs, is part of responsible sexuality. This is done by making an appointment with your doctor (or local sexual health center) to discuss birth control, tests, treatment for sexually transmitted infections, and other information about your sexual health.

If you find out after being tested that you have an STI, it is very important to avoid accusing, blaming, or ruining others' reputations. Some people make bad choices, but catching something is not uncommon, and many infections do not have clear signs and symptoms, so they can be passed from person to person without carriers knowing they are doing so. If other people were cool enough to let you see them naked and do fun things with them, then it is the polite thing to do to give them the benefit of the doubt and a little respect until you are sure.

It is also very important to let any partners you've had since your last testing know you have an STI. If you have (or even suspect you may have) an STI of any kind, you must tell your sexual partners before your pants come off! Failing to tell previous partners that they may have been exposed to something not only jeopardizes their health, but also could lead to them infecting others (and it makes you look like a jerk).

Call the American Pregnancy Helpline (866-942-6466, thehelpline. org) or Planned Parenthood (800-230-PLAN (7526), plannedparent-hood.org) where help, support, and information are available twenty-four hours a day, seven days a week.

# SEXUAL HEALTH

There are seven crucial criteria that need to be met in order for a sexual interaction to be considered responsible.

## The Seven Crucial Criteria of a Responsible Sexual Interaction[1]

1. Privacy

2. Consent

3. Age appropriateness

4. Foreplay

5. Safer sex

6. Afterplay

7. The Big R's

### Privacy

Despite our culture's love of reality TV, a lot of people get squicked out when they see people having sex in public. Plus, it's illegal almost everywhere.

## Consent

Consent can be defined as an informed, mutual, sober, honest, understood, and revisited agreement. It is both persons' responsibility to give and obtain clear consent.

*The Rules of Consent*[2]

**Consent must be informed.** Terms like "hook up," "sex," and "doing it" mean different things to different people. If you can't talk about it, you shouldn't be doing it.

**Consent must be mutual.** Equality is key. People too far below your age range, development, mentality, or authority level cannot legally give consent.

**Consent must be sober.** If you are too drunk to drive a car, you are too drunk to drive your genitals.[3] Drunk, high, or sleeping people can't give consent.

**Consent must be honest.** True consent cannot be manipulated. A "yes" after twenty minutes of whining, guilting, bugging, or begging is not actually a "yes."

---

### LGBTW . . . Sex and Substances

Drugs and alcohol are designed to disinhibit—suppressing the parts of the brain that control judgment. This means that substances can (and often do) allow people to make different choices than they would if they were sober.

Mixing sex and substances is problematic in several ways:

- Safer sex techniques can be done incorrectly or forgotten altogether.

- Communication can be confused or not done at all.

- Decision-making can become compromised.

- People can pressure or be pressured into activities or situations they were not anticipating or comfortable with.

- Consent is not able to be given or received while under the influence of substances.

---

**Consent must be understood.** Consent is not just about getting a "yes." Consent also means people get to say "no." The absence of "no" does not mean the answer is "yes." If you are unsure, ask. When you say "no," say it clearly; no "ums" and no giggling.

**Consent must be revisited.** Consent is a process, not a goal. For the next level, the next day, the next date . . . you and they need to ask again. Giving consent once does not mean you can't say "no" later. Even if you are in a relationship with someone or you've let them do stuff before, they still need to ask each time. People get to say "no" anytime—even if they've already said "yes."

Bottom line: it is illegal—not to mention unethical and reprehensible—to have sex without consent.

## Age Appropriateness

The state or region in which you live most likely has specific guidelines on the age of consent. It is wise to be aware of these before you choose to engage in sexual activity. (It is also a good idea to research the laws of other states, regions, and countries when you move or are traveling, because nothing can ruin that trip to New York, your freshman year in college, that semester in Italy, or summer at Grandma's beach house like a felony.)

For those of you still in high school, here are good general guidelines:

- Limit all sexual activities to people within two years of your own age.

- Limit your sexual activities to non-penetrative acts until age sixteen.

- Reserve "varsity level" sex acts for people whom you know well, have ongoing caring feelings for, who are willing, and who are insistent on safer-sex practices.

Once you are older than the age of eighteen, **"the age rule"** kicks in and will be applicable for the rest of your life:

- Take your age.

- Divide it in half.

- Add nine.

- Do not have sex with people younger than the number you come up with.

This simple equation will help to ensure that you engage in sexual/romantic relationships with people in your general cohort. As we get older, age differences become less important. For example, a forty-two-year-old's and a thirty-eight-year-old's lives probably don't look that different. Likewise, a twenty-nine-year-old and a twenty-six-year-old are probably going through the same general life stages. However, a twenty-two-year-old's and a twenty-year-old's lives should look and feel very different. Even a nineteen-year-old and an eighteen-year-old—even though they may be only one year apart in age—are potentially living very different lives, especially if one has graduated, moved out of their parents' house or started college, while the other is still in high school.

*Note*: Though it can be tempting to be vague or less than honest about your age when dating other people, it can cause a lot of problems. When a younger person lies about their age and gets involved with an older person, it is the older person who can get into massive trouble, including legal charges. Be cool and don't risk anyone else's reputation or freedom by not being yourself.

## Foreplay

Foreplay is important for getting your partner ready for sex. Foreplay is all the fun, kind-of-romantic, sort-of-intimate stuff people do before they have sex. Some people consider the kissing and cuddling and other parts of foreplay just as important as the actual sex.

## Safer Sex

Safer sex is on this list for obvious reasons; sex cannot be considered responsible without safer-sex methods firmly in place.

## Afterplay

Afterplay is all the fun, kind-of-romantic, sort-of-intimate stuff people do after they have sex. This is important for communication, connection, and caring . . . and, sometimes, can make the difference between having sex with someone again or not.

## The Big R's

These are respect, relationship, and reciprocation. Sexual morality is not about when you are allowed to have sex; it is about how you treat people when you are in sexual contact with them.

There is no realistic way to make a list of rules that will apply and be useful to all people in all situations, cultures, times, or places. This is why it is important to act with **respect**.

Many of you will have sex with someone along the way that you are not in love with. But as long as you have some kind of **relationship** with them, that might be OK. Hookups and lifelong partnerships happen, but if one partner is having a one-night stand, but the other thinks it is the beginning of something bigger, that is a problem.

**Reciprocity** is another word for balance or fairness. This is about both people investing in the relationship in approximately the same amount without the pressure or awkwardness of a power differential, such as a boss/employee, teacher/student, or coach/athlete situation. Imbalances such as those are what make sexual relationships less-than-healthy and sometimes, illegal. Reciprocity also has to do with making sure that both people are participating and enjoying the sex. If you are wanting someone to give you oral sex, for example, you should be willing to do the same for them.

The Big R's look different to different people in different situations, at different times, and in different cultures. Morality is relative. That means what is OK for some people, in some places, at some times is not OK for, in, or at others.

- Do you cheat?

- Do you have sex with someone who is cheating on someone else?

- Do you tell someone if you have an STI?

- Do you go out with or have sex with someone when it clearly means something more to them than it does to you?

173

- Do you lie about your age or experience?
- Do you hook up with someone who is drunk?

The bottom line is that in order to go at sexual and intimate interactions respectfully, you must

- act in a way that you would want to be treated,
- err on the side of caution,
- avoid knowingly or accidentally doing something that could, would, or might harm someone (including yourself).

# PART SEVEN
# "DON'T LEAVE ME THIS WAY"

As I acknowledged in the beginning of this book, queer people are stronger than others due to our struggles, more creative due to having to think outside larger, cultural boxes, and braver in the face of both external adversity and our own inner journeys.

As with other minorities, hate crimes and bias will come and go in waves, though will likely always be a looming feature of life. LGBT people face adversity, invisibility, and violence every day, just because we exist.

Though the world is populated with so many opportunities, so much encouragement, safe spaces, and reasons to show pride, we must also remember that predators and haters are real, as are the problems and barriers they will try to create.

It is up to you to do what you can to change that dynamic, but also to prepare for it, to do what you can to protect yourself and those around you, and to persist with pride while you are doing so.

## CHAPTER TWENTY-FOUR
# SEXUAL HARM

Sexual and gender minorities (like all minorities) have always been targets for fear and prejudice. These biases are perpetuated (and sometimes created) by the now-classic myths about LGBT people.

These myths include: gay men molest children; trans people will rape you in the bathroom; you can "catch," choose, or unturn gay; being trans is a mental health issue; supporting hate crime laws will somehow lead to the legalization of bestiality or child sexual abuse; and granting someone else certain rights will lessen the amount of rights for others—like they are french fries or something, not freedoms we can all share.

Part of this lies in the dark roots of queerphobia in that—unlike other minority populations—queer people and issues trigger the fear that some cis/straight people have about their own, not-necessarily rigid sexuality. For example, someone may hate Jewish or Muslim people or be afraid of a black or Latino person, but they don't have an unconscious, deep-seated fear that they may someday convert unwillingly to another religion, or are secretly on some level a person of a different color. But there are those in the world

- who have gay thoughts and feelings from time to time,

- who have had a sexual dream about a same sex friend or celebrity,

- who have had same sex experiences and are ashamed because of messages they have received from their families,

- who have been molested by someone of the same sex, and believe that was the cause of the abuser's violence or

- are actually, legitimately queer though think they must remain closeted.

Sometimes these people do not have the ego strength to put those ideas into context, to explore their thoughts and feelings, or accept the reality of their lives. They remain closed off, focused on their emotional and nonsensical beliefs, and turn their frustration, anger, and fear on others who represent what they themselves fear most.

These anti-gay/anti-trans myths are easily debunked by virtually all legitimate medical and scientific authority, though their presence contributes to the reality that GLBT people are more targeted for hate crime violence than any other community.[1]

When one thinks that large chunks of the population are illegitimate, threatening, or "less-than," it is easier to turn down your humanity and do harm to that population, including sexual harm—sexual assault, child sexual abuse, and harassment.

# HARASSMENT, ABUSE, AND ASSAULT

Sexual harassment can be defined as any unwelcome sexualized attention. It can include a range of behaviors, from inappropriate behaviors and annoyances to serious abuses. Despite what many people believe, sexual harassment is not limited to forced sexual activity.[1]

Sexual harassment can be

- verbal like talking to (or at) someone in a sexual way or making crude comments or jokes,

- digital such as posting or sharing sexual comments or photos, or

- physical such as failing to get (or ignoring) consent.

Sexual harassment can also involve making the environments we learn, work, live, and play in uncomfortable for others in a sexual way. Lewd comments and jokes, sexual teasing, or spreading sexual stories about a classmate or workmate, inappropriately directed flirting and/or pervasively sexualized overtones, especially in groups or when there is a perceived power or cultural differential, can all be perceived as offensive, degrading, or intimidating.

If someone else is making you feel uncomfortable or is harassing you in your school or workplace, say something—if not to the perpetrator, then to a teacher, a parent, or manager.

Likewise, remember that behaving in a way that others perceive as harassing can bring serious consequences. Pay attention to how you treat others, and how those others react to you.

Child sexual abuse can be defined as a violation of trust in a relationship with any or all of the following characteristics:

- unequal power and/or advanced knowledge

- the need for secrecy

- sexualized activity (*sexualized*, not necessarily sexual)[2]

Whenever one person dominates and exploits a younger person through sexual activity or suggestion, or uses sexual feelings and behavior to degrade, humiliate, control, injure, or misuse the other person, it qualifies as sexual abuse.[3] Sexual abuse can include violations of a position of trust, power, and protection against those who lack an adequately developed emotional, or intellectual "immune system," and it promotes sexual secrecy among the people who are victimized.

Sexual abuse involves direct touching, fondling, and/or intercourse against a person's will.[4] Examples include kissing; oral sex; penetration with objects, genitals, or fingers; and masturbation. Use of force is sometimes involved, though this does not mean it is always physical or violent.

Sexual abuse frequently occurs in the context of a relationship. This can be family (such as an older sibling or parental figure), but can also happen in teacher-student, coach-athlete, and boss-employee relationships. Sexual abuse is about an unfair balance of power, most often an age difference, but can also involve differences in physical power, emotional power, intellectual power, or social power, along with numerous manipulative techniques such as secrecy, bribery, trickery, lies, and threats.

**Sexual abuse**

- often causes negative feelings, such as confusion, fear, anger, shame, depression, and worthlessness;

- can potentially cause positive feelings, such as feeling special, appreciated, noticed, and loved, as well as physical pleasure;

- is not necessarily violent. Exposure to pornography, for example, can be considered sexual abuse;

- can be hands on (for example, kissing, touching, penetration) or hands off (such as exposure to sexual body parts or acts, being watched or photographed in vulnerable situations).

The prevalence of childhood sexual abuse is remarkably high for both boys and girls. According to the National Center for Missing and Exploited Children, 20 percent of all children are molested before the age of eighteen.[5] Most abuse occurs prior to age sixteen; almost two-thirds occurs before the age of twelve; more than half of that before age six.[6]

**In fact, out of every one hundred friends you have on Facebook, Instagram, or Snapchat, more than forty will (statistically) be survivors of sexual abuse.**[7]

Examples of the traumatic effects of abuse include

- anxiety/panic attacks
- depression
- distractibility/difficulty concentrating
- guilt/shame
- insomnia
- intimacy issues/loss of trust
- irritability/anger
- loss of self-esteem
- memory loss
- negative body image/eating disorders
- nightmares/flashbacks
- numbness/apathy
- poor choice in future partners/victim mentality
- promiscuity
- self-mutilation/harm

- sexual dysfunction

- shock/denial

- social withdrawal/isolation

- substance abuse

- suicidal ideation/attempts

A child who is abused or made to do sexual things with an adult is never to blame—even if they consented to the abuse at the time, cared about their abuser, or enjoyed parts of it. Sexual acts during sex offenses are *not* sex. They are abuse.

Sexual harassment (typically verbal or technological) and abuse (typically referring to the victimization of children) are subcategories of the larger concept of sexual assault. Sexual assault is an umbrella term that involves non-consensual sexual contact and unwanted sexual activity toward anyone regardless of age, gender, or orientation.[8]

Sexual contact of any kind without that person's consent is considered sexual assault.

People who commit assault can be acquaintances, family members, coworkers, or friends. When this happens in an established relationship it is referred to as date rape, but sexual assault also happens when the abused and the abuser do not know each other at all.

Sexual assault can

- involve penetration or touching.

- happen while nude or while clothed.

- range from fondling and kissing, to being forced to perform or receive vaginal, anal, or oral sex.

- include sexually explicit material—being forced or tricked into viewing or creating sexually explicit pictures or video, or sharing consensual images non-consensually.

- involve a health care professional, teacher, coach, or some other person in authority touching your body in an unprofessional, unwarranted, and inappropriate manner.

Sexually assaultive behavior can involve physical acts or happen in the form of exposure by forcing someone to view sexually explicit images or acts. *Any* unwanted or non-consensual touch that causes that person to feel uncomfortable, hurt, or scared is illegal and can be considered sexual assault.

Abusers typically break other people's boundaries through manipulation. When someone does something someone likes in order to get them to go along with unwanted sexual contact, it is called grooming. This can include bribes or special favors. When someone does something someone does not like in order to get them to go along with it, it is called coercion. This can involve things like tricks, blackmail, and other threats. Manipulation can also involve violence and physically forcing someone into sexual contact.

---

## LGBTW . . . Date Rape Drugs[9]

Date-rape drugs are chemicals that can be put into your drink that weaken you and impair your ability to move or remember things.

There are three main kinds of date-rape drugs:

- gamma-hydroxybutyrate (GHB)

- Rohypnol, also called rophys (pronounced "roofies")

- ketamine hydrochloride[10]

These drugs are typically colorless and odorless, and can be easily slipped into drinks, such as soda or alcohol, without being detected.

When you are in social or public situations with people you do not know:

- Do not accept drinks that are handed to you by someone you don't know well (unless you watched it being made).

- Don't leave your drink unattended. If you must leave it, leave it with a trusted friend (emphasis on *trusted*), or get a new one when you come back.

- Be aware of your surroundings and trust your gut—when people hear about "Date Rape Drugs" they think about alcoholic drinks

---

- at frat parties or in bars being spiked, but *any* drink, alcoholic or not, can be tampered with.

**If you taste or see anything strange in any drink, or begin to feel strange:**

- Stop drinking immediately.

- Let someone nearby know what you suspect has happened (these chemicals can begin working very quickly).

- Ask them to call the police.

At some point, someone may offer you one of these for recreational use or because "it's fun" or "makes sex better." Don't do it. These are sedative and hypnotic drugs that are used during medical procedures, not recreational drugs.

Typically sexual contact crosses legal lines if one of the parties involved was pressured, threatened, forced, intoxicated, unconscious or if there was a power differential between the two people such as age, development, or mental ability.

Sexual assault is traumatic and every person's response to that trauma can be different. Some people can recover quickly, while others can be quite traumatized in lasting ways. Factors that influence this can include the frequency (how often it happened), the intensity (the level of violence and injury), and the duration (how long it went on) of the assaults.[11] Other factors that can impact how traumatized someone is and how quickly they recover from sexual assault include

- how old someone was when they were abused,

- their relationship to the abuser, and

- the responses from their support systems—including police, health professionals, friends, and (especially) parents.

**If you or someone you know experience any unwanted sexual contact:**

- Tell someone who cares—a parent, friend, teacher, etc.

- Get medical attention to check for infections or other injuries.

- Call the police.

- Call the National Sexual Assault Hotline, (800) 656-HOPE (4673).

The National Sexual Assault Hotline is hosted by RAINN (the Rape, Abuse and Incest National Network). Based on your zip code or the first six numbers of your phone, you will be connected to free, RAINN-affiliated, sexual assault resources in your area, where you can find and access:

- confidential support from a trained staff member to help you talk through what happened

- information about the laws and legal services in your area

- basic information about medical concerns, and locations for health facilities for everything from emergency response to first aid to physical examination and testing

- contacts for other local resources that can assist with your next steps toward help, healing and recovery, and reporting

*Note:* The decision about whether or not to press charges against someone who has sexually assaulted you can wait, but necessary evidence may need to be collected immediately. If charges might be pressed, then not bathing, and not changing clothes or even washing your hands can be helpful. Writing down everything you can remember and keeping any evidence such as items with the offender's DNA on it or any digital communications is a good idea as well.

Seeking medical attention and alerting the authorities are high up on the list of self-care following any kind of sexual assault. But the most important thing is to tell someone. Sexual assault touches everyone's life, and anyone can be victimized, but if we surround ourselves with supportive people—both personal and professional—the effects can be lessened.

## CHAPTER TWENTY-SIX
# PERSONAL SAFETY

I n light of the fact that far too many people are assaulted physically and sexually in this country:

- Understand that most people who are sexually victimized know their attackers.[1]

- Acknowledge how your gender or sexual orientation and expression may make you a target.

- Be aware of the very real possibility that at some point in your life, someone will try to seriously harm you in some way.

- Work to build strong instincts and boundaries.

- Self-defense classes are a really good idea for everyone.

**Things you can do to keep yourself safe and lessen the chances of being victimized:**

- Be aware that walking alone at night may be dangerous.

- Observe constantly. Do not engage in behaviors that restrict your observation.

- Walk with your head up and a confident stride, and don't let your listening devices completely restrict your hearing.

- Stay in well-lit areas.

- Trust your gut. If something feels weird, it probably is.

- Know your routes. Notice lighting, alleys, abandoned buildings, and street people.

- Try to vary your routine. Don't let your behavior be too predictable and avoid walking the same path at the same time each time.

- If you are alone and worry that you are being followed (or you see a person or group farther down the street that makes you feel uncomfortable), cross the street, walk in another direction, or ask other people walking if you can stay with them for a while.

- When walking to your door or apartment, carry your keys in your hand, ready to use.

- While waiting for public transportation, keep your back against a wall (or pole) so that you cannot be surprised from behind.

- Elevators are safer than stairs, but trust your gut if you are alone and there is someone else in the elevator.

- When parking your car, note its location carefully so that you can go directly to it.

- When returning to your car, look around. If you notice anything or anyone suspicious, go back the way you came.

- If you have electric locks, know how to unlock the driver's door only (as opposed to all the doors at the same time).

- If you return to your car and find it parked next to a big van—especially one without side windows—enter your car from the passenger door, or wait and come back later.

- Do not park next to big vans—especially those without side windows.

- As soon as you get into your car, lock the doors and leave.

- If you run out of gas or have an accident, don't take rides from strangers. If a stranger wants to help, ask that person to call a repair truck or police officer for you (if you haven't already).

- But strive to keep your gas tank and your phone battery as full as possible.

- If you see an accident or a stranded motorist and you are alone, it is probably more helpful to call 911 on your cell phone than to stop.

- Do not allow strangers into your car.

- Do not allow strangers into your home.

- Never go outside to investigate a strange noise (we've all seen that movie).

- Always let someone know where you are going, what you are doing, who you will be with, and when you will be back—especially for trips, parties, first dates, and similar situations. This is especially important when meeting an online date for the first time.

- When first getting to know someone, keep your dates in public places, such as restaurants, malls, or theaters.

- Group dates are also great when you first start getting to know someone.

- Travel in groups as often as possible, especially when going to parties or clubs.

- Contract with friends to stay (and leave) together.

- Don't break those contracts.

- Understand your limitations around substances, and realize how much they can increase your risk of having something bad happen.

- Do not leave food or drink unattended when you go to the bathroom.

## LGBTW . . . Peeing (Yes, We're Still Talking About This)

In 2016, the US Departments of Education and Justice under the Obama Administration made it clear that those who identify as a particular sex can use the restroom that applies to them.[2]

Schools were told that they should allow trans students to use the restroom that aligns with their gender identification, under an educational amendment from 1972, called Title IX (nine), which banned discrimination on the basis of sex. The Obama Administration, logically and humanely, suggested that Title IX includes discrimination on the basis of gender identity as well. Schools were instructed to set up separate locker-room/restroom areas if they chose to. These areas could be offered as an option to everyone, but no one in particular would be ordered to use them.[3]

Because of this, some states are in the process of suing the government to keep trans people from using the appropriate restrooms—not only in schools but in other public areas as well. In addition (at the time of this writing) the Trump Administration has reversed those policy recommendations, and threatened to cut federal funding to schools that continue to allow students to use the restroom that aligns with their gender.

Arguments of the people opposed to gender neutral and aligned bathrooms include:

- Some vague idea of public safety being threatened. Some are arguing that men will suddenly dress as women in order to infiltrate women's restrooms to sexually assault them. This argument is particularly silly in that (as of the time of this writing) there is zero documentation of any trans person ever having sexually assaulted someone in a public restroom.[4] What these laws are ironically protesting are the dangers that straight men (not trans women) pose to people in the women's restrooms.

- Some, again vague, idea of an encroachment of some people's freedoms. It's the same argument that has been used against "gay" marriage; as if gay people get married, then there won't be enough marriage left for straight people (?), or maybe their straight marriages won't be "marriagey" enough anymore (?!). . . . It's as if their arguments have started driving before their brains have put their seat belts on.

These arguments make zero sense when you think about them rationally. They are cruel and rife with misunderstandings about trans issues that are hateful, unacceptable, and just not rooted in reality. This (and issues like it) will be ongoing, but we will get them sorted eventually.

The reality is that trans and non-binary people have been peeing in public restrooms since they were invented, and no one has noticed or cared.

Culturally, The Gay Conversation has been going on for several decades now, and people are finally wising and warming up, but The Gender Conversation is happening much more quickly and much more loudly.

Gender doesn't separate cleanly into two categories the way a lot of people (for a long time) thought it did. There are more flavors of people than there used to be, and different ways in which people's gender identity doesn't match up with their sex in necessarily expected or easy-to-understand ways.

Gender is fluid and mutable and that concept can be *very* confusing to people who haven't had to deal with it before, to people who don't encounter it on a regular basis, to people who are afraid or isolated or just simply ignorant. There are a *lot* of people who fall into those categories, and (though they need to acknowledge that gender isn't just about penises and vaginas anymore and get over it) the rest of us need to acknowledge that this is new, and that they should be treated with a degree of compassion.

Bottom line:

- Pee when and where it makes sense for you.

- Go with confidence (no pun intended)—you have every right to be there, so act like it.

- Do your best to not make anyone uncomfortable.

- Don't put up with others trying to make you feel uncomfortable.

- Use words not violence when you do this (*Note*: this is harder to do if you have testosterone in your system).

- If you are treated negatively by someone while entering, inside, or leaving, leave the situation and call security.

- If you are treated negatively by an employee while entering, inside, or leaving, ask for their name, then find their manager.

- The crowdsourcing review site/app, Yelp, now provides the ability to list and find businesses that have non-gender-specific restrooms—typically private, locking restrooms that are open to people of all genders.

- For those who prefer private restrooms, Starbucks are *everywhere*, and not only provide delicious, caffeinated beverages, but also single occupancy bathrooms.

- Above all, be safe and smart. Use situational awareness—stay aware of your surroundings and context, and if you have the sense that a particular bathroom choice is going to bring down violence upon you, then consider your options. You are *not* Rosa Parks; it is as ridiculous and unnecessary for you to make one, particular toilet stall *so* important that you actively invite someone else's violence as it is ridiculous and unnecessary for the haters to make that same stall so important that it justifies their violence. Live to pee another day.

- And don't forget to wash your hands.

**If you are attacked:**

- If you can, run.

- If you run, run loudly!

- If you are attacked and there is no safe alternative (like running), then decide to defend yourself and do it immediately.

- Take the fight to them. Cut off their attack and incapacitate them.

- Do this loudly, too.

- The elbow is the strongest point in your body. If you are close enough to use it, use it.

- Go for the squishy parts: eyes and balls. Try to take out their vision and/or wind.

- Strike with total disregard for their safety.

- Never regret anything you do to save your own life.

**Things you can do to lessen the chances of other people being victimized:**

**Always watch each other's backs.** Never stand by the abuse of another—particularly those who have a minority status (sexual or not).

Whether or not you are ever targeted directly for harassment or assault, work to find ways to participate in activism: joining or creating gay-straight alliances, or advocating to change school policies and even laws. **Activism helps—not just you, but everyone else as well**.

# PART EIGHT
## "I WILL SURVIVE"

There will be people in your life who cannot handle your LGBTQ-ness. Homophobia. Biphobia. Transphobia. Just-Being-Chill-About-It-Phobia—Whatever-The-Phobia. They all suck. But they are real. Be ready for it. Some of them will be friends, some will be family. Some will be people who hire you or fire you. Some will be neighbors. Some will be classmates. Some will be your elected officials who supposedly represent you. Some will be behind you in line while shopping, at the movies, or boarding a plane. Some will be behind the counter.

Some will make snarky comments barely loud enough for you to hear as you walk past, some will say nothing to your face (but plenty to others), some will say nothing but speak volumes with their stares, others will step up and say actively hateful things right to your face.

Why people do this (and how you handle it) may vary greatly, but it is very important that you remember:

- It is not about you. It's about them.

- It will still feel like it's about you.

- A percentage of them will come around.

- It will not necessarily be the ones that you need to come around.

- It will not be enough of them.

- It will get better.

## CHAPTER TWENTY-SEVEN
# SEXUALIZED HARM

Unfortunately, it is still important to consider your safety when thinking about what to do on a date. Ideally, you'd be able to go anywhere at any time and kiss or hold hands with your date at the movies, the park, walking down the street, or at the school dance. However, if you know your classmates or larger community lean homophobic, PDA (public displays of affection) may not be the smartest or safest idea. This is obviously not OK, but it can be the reality depending on your setting and circumstance. Your safety (and that of your date) is the most important thing, and it is important to use situational awareness to balance out the political and social benefits of being free and expressive with that safety in the face of potential violence.

Most people experience bullying and harassment at some point. This is even more common for queer and gender expansive kids, though a major difference is that (different than straight/cis kids) much of even the non-sexual harassment that queer kids have to deal with is still about their sexuality or identity. It's not technically sexual harassment, but it is sexualized. . . .

When's the last time you saw a kid made fun of because she was straight?

How often do you hear about a kid being threatened because he was being too-cis? (There's even the derogatory term, "sissy," but that is *not* what it means!)

If you find yourself being targeted and harassed because of your sex, gender, orientation, or expression:

- Find respect and allies in supportive peers and family.

If you think they may not be trying to be jerks, but maybe just being clod-dish or ignorant,

- Use your words—an assertive conversation may help change their behavior and/or encourage them to choose their words differently.

If they are clearly trying to get a rise and reaction from you,

- Ignore them.

---

## LGBTW . . . Homodium

The term "homophobia" was introduced by psychologist George Weinberg in 1967[1] to refer to people with apprehension about homosexuality and homosexual people. Those apprehensions mostly involved fear and igno-rance of queer people and dynamics. A phobia is generally considered an irrational fear of something.

There has been ignorance (and because of that, fear) of queer people for as long as there have been people. Eventually, through science, pop culture, technology, and shifts in our social landscape, homophobia came to be generally considered a "bad thing."

It has come to be widely used and a generalized term for a range of negative attitudes toward queer or non-straight/cis experiences or people (or both). Since the Internet happened, even more specific terms such as biphobic and transphobia have surfaced.

Though not an actual, mental disorder, homophobia is considered a negative character trait, an attitude or personality flaw that can be balanced out and shifted by education, or relationships with and exposure to queer people and experiences. The more someone learns about homosexuality, and the more people come out (both as queer and as allies), the easier it is for that person to move from homophobia to tolerance and even active support.

Dr. Weinberg also acknowledged that fear and phobias can "lead to great brutality, as fear always does."[2]

And there has been great brutality. Social, emotional, and, of course, physical brutality against queer people. But sometimes this is not always fear-based.

It is understandable that a chunk of the human population may have a hard time developing a relationship with complex concepts such as sex and gender, expression, and identity. Queer people can still be expected to find empathy for people who have not caught up yet, who may be struggling to catch up and just don't quite get it, or who are actively working to change ingrained preconceptions.

That being said, opposition, aversion, horror, and hatred of queer people, queer experience (and arguably even queer existence) has been fueled, and perpetuated and allowed by certain current world leaders. These leaders have given voice and legitimacy to hateful and outdated attitudes that have not been socially acceptable for a very long time, with Putin (Russia), Johnson (England), and, of course, Trump (America) being the primary offenders.

If one has the access to information, the opportunity to learn, and the capacity to understand and is *still* able to muster up the energy to injure or oppress someone who is different—*that* is true bigotry. That is not about being afraid. That is intended and targeted hatred and chosen disgust.

And the Latin root of hatred or disgust is odium,[3] not phobos.

As Dr. Weinberg pointed out, the brutality (the hateful and violent actions) comes from the fear, but they are different things. Homophobia and homodium are different things.

There are people who may be truly homophobic—those who are very young, very isolated, perhaps very old . . . education and experience can counterbalance legitimate gaps in understanding and exposure.

Ignorance is not stupidity. Ignorance is a lack of information. Ignorance is understandable. Not handling ignorance is not an excuse—it's **homodium**.

Homodic behavior is different than simply not getting it. It's having the exposure, the opportunity for experience, and the ability to understand something different than your own experience and *not* doing that.

The homodipaths who purposely create and perpetuate the violence and oppression are different than your elderly aunt who says something stupid at Thanksgiving dinner.

This current wave of oppression and fueled hatred against LGBT people, the permission given to established hate groups, the open insults and the political actions against GLBT individuals and their basic rights and dignity (sometimes, jokingly called Gaycism) can no longer be considered simply homophobic. Those behaviors aren't leading to the brutality. They *are* the brutality.

You will encounter those who fear or do not understand you. The healthy and appropriate response to this is connection, patience, and information. You will also encounter people who do not want to understand you and who hate, rather than fear you. The healthiest and safest approach in those situations is protecting yourselves (and others) through actions, activism, and resources.

## CHAPTER TWENTY-EIGHT
# COPING WITH MINORITY STRESS

M inority Stress is the particular flavor of stress experienced by members of marginalized and stigmatized minority groups. These groups can be identified and categorized by race, ethnicity, socioeconomic status, and gender and sexuality.

## Stress Responses

People in minority groups who experience high levels of prejudice, discrimination, social stigma, harassment, violence, rejection, and/or the denial of basic rights and oppression develop stress responses that grow stronger over time. These responses lead to social, mental, and physical problems.[1]

For GLBT people, these problems show up as

- being/staying closeted.

- internalized homo/trans phobia.

- higher levels of rejection sensitivity (expecting rejection).

- lower levels of assertiveness and making fewer healthy choices.

These things lead to other negative outcomes such as:

### Dropping Out of School

LGBT students are statistically twice as likely to not plan on completing high school or going on to college than straight/cis kids.[2]

## Substance Abuse

Between 20 percent and 30 percent of GLBT people abuse substances, compared to about 9 percent of the general population.[3]

## Homelessness

Approximately 40 percent of all American homeless youth identify as LGBTQ—most of whom have been disowned by someone.[4]

## Survival Sex (Trading Sex for Money, Food or Shelter)

Almost half of young homeless people of all sexual orientations have traded sex because they had no place to stay.[5]

## Mental Health Issues

GLBT individuals are almost three times more likely than others to experience major depression or generalized anxiety disorder.

## Suicide

For LGBTQ people aged ten to twenty-four, suicide is the leading cause of death.[6] GLBT youth are four times more likely to attempt suicide than straight people the same age.[7] Worse still, when a gay kid attempts suicide, they are four times more likely to give themselves a life-threatening injury than their straight counterparts.[8] If you identify with more than one minority (such as being gay *and* homeless, or being trans *and* black), the volume on the minority stress can be turned up even higher.[9]

# Dealing with Minority Stress

There are many common techniques that people use to deal with everyday life stressors, including:

- Exercise.

- Healthy eating habits.

- Avoiding drugs, alcohol, marijuana, and tobacco.

- Paying attention to your body's limits around caffeine.

- Task and goal management.

- Assertive (as opposed to aggressive or passive) communication.

- Muscle relaxation exercises and abdominal breathing.

- Meditation.

- Art and journaling.

- Avoiding perfectionism. (Being "excellent" is a much more realistic and attainable goal!)

- Replacing negative self-talk with more positive thoughts.

- Building a network of people who help and support you.

- Helping and supporting others.

Specifically, through coming out, LGBT people can learn to cope with and overcome the adverse effects of stress.[10]

Being out can help queer minorities counteract stress by establishing an identity to a larger network of other out people with structures, traditions, and values. People can come to understand that there are places they belong and groups that will embrace them, even if some others do not.

Along those same lines, it is true that queer prejudice and violence can lead to trauma and negative outcomes for individual people, but through things such as activism, pride, and self-acceptance, those same traumas can become opportunities for growth and motivation to help and support others—which can balance out and even improve physical and mental health outcomes.[11,12]

---

## LGBTW . . . Pride (with a capital P)

The birth of the modern Pride movement was the Stonewall Riots.[13,14] In the middle of the larger civil rights movements and during a raid in The Stonewall Inn—a popular gay bar in Greenwich Village in New York—the crowd of queer patrons began to resist and ultimately demonstrate against unfair and inappropriate targeting by the police.

At the time the US government and police departments around the country kept lists of known homosexuals. Laws were put in place to keep LGBT people out of parks, restaurants, and schools. Bars and clubs catering to them were shut down, universities expelled instructors suspected of being homosexual, and cross-dressing was illegal. Thousands of GLBTQ men and women were publicly humiliated, physically harassed, fired, jailed, or institutionalized in mental hospitals.

Around 2:00 a.m. on Saturday, June 28, 1969, police raided The Stonewall Inn, a then-non-descript bar in Manhattan. During the seize, patrons were threatened with outing and violence, and trans customers were shuttled to a back room and forced to show their genitals as proof of their gender—some were sexually assaulted and harassed as well.

But those who escaped (before the windows were boarded) or were allowed to leave didn't run. They stopped outside. This was pre–social media, but word spread quickly through the neighborhood, then the city, and the customers of the inn were soon joined by dozens of other queer men and women and their allies.

The crowd grew angry and resistant and larger. Their demonstration went on for hours, was even larger the next day with protesters numbering over a thousand, and (though it was eventually dispersed by a riot-control squad), things were never quite the same.

Demonstrations continued for days after the riot at Stonewall, spreading throughout the city of New York.

Celebrations honoring the anniversary of the first public demonstrations for LGBT rights gradually spread across the country, and now there are worldwide Pride events during the month of June.

Today, celebrating Pride represents something different for everyone: joy, unity, rebellion, fairness, freedom, connection, the opposite of the shame that so many others try to associate with being queer.

Some think that it is just about rainbow flags, drag queens, and glitter. Yes, music, food, games, entertainers, and loads of people wearing (and not wearing) fabulous costumes and outfits are a big part of it, but there are political, educational, and outreach aspects to modern Pride celebrations as well.

Some think it's about acting gay or feeling queer or being trans, but on a very real level it isn't about that at all.

- It's about acting however-you-want-without-having-to-be-self-conscious.

- It's about feeling human—just like everyone else.

- It's about being You without having to hide, censor, or pretend.

Surrounded by others just like you, you can just act/feel/be *You*. (And there *are* rainbow flags, drag queens, and glitter.)

## LGBTW . . . Activism

Working with other people and groups in your community to motivate political and social change is important.

- Because there is safety in numbers, and joining together makes everyone safer.

- Because it's not just about you. As hard as it can be to be queer right now, it was harder yesterday. Others have made sacrifices and changes before you so that it is easier for you than it was for them. It's important to pay it forward.

- Because there is a lot of hate out there. It is fueled by politics, religions, and media, and when smart, caring, and healthy people band together to balance that out, the scales tip, and that narrative changes just a bit.

- Because there is a lot of stupid out there. It is fueled by politics, religions, and media, and when smart, caring, and healthy people band together to balance that out, the scales tip, and that narrative changes just a bit.

- Because Matthew Shepard.

- Because Orlando.

- Because It Gets Better.

Queer people can address violent crime against the GLBT community by

- Using social media.
- Joining a local neighborhood watch program.
- Working with their local police department's LGBTQ liaison.
- Reporting crimes and encouraging others to do the same.
- Volunteering to help repair acts of vandalism.
- Attending vigils, protests, and rallies.
- Get involved and suggest some action from your friends, school, club, team, or house of worship.

## LGBTW . . . School

**Stay. In. School.**

It is super important to get the best possible education you can. This will:

- Increase your chances of a job with health benefits that match your unique needs.
- Earn you money for self-sufficiency.
- Expose you to more educated (and likely liberal) people.

Bottom line: **Having a good education will give you more options in life.**

At school:

- Develop good study habits.
- Stay physically active.
- Make some friends. Stay socially active. Join a club or two.
- Try not to make enemies. Be kind, cool, and classy to everyone. Smile.

- Find resources and connections outside of school.

- Find opportunities to volunteer (if your school doesn't have a GSA/QSA, start one!). Make a difference in the world.

If school becomes absolutely unsafe or unbearable (that happens sometimes), online school can be an option. There are also high school completion courses offered at some community colleges as well as G.E.D. classes—these can get you past the high school thing. Meanwhile, you can focus on college and/or get a job, and start making some down-the-road goals.

## LGBTW . . . Suicide

- Do not turn someone else's hatred, fear, or issues on yourself. You will encounter enough enemies in life—they do not need your help.

- Do not respond to someone else's hatred, fear, or issues by creating your own.

- Do not respond to someone else's violence with violence—we do not fight monsters by becoming them.

- When you do feel hatred and fear, try to channel it into something productive (see above re: activism).

- Harming yourself is not the response to have in the face of someone else's Whatever-The-Phobia.

- Show them they are wrong.

- Do your best to avoid them when you can't.

- Do your best to feel bad for them when you can't avoid them.

- And always, always reach out for help.

**If you are having thoughts about wanting to die:**

Call the National Teen Suicide Hotline (866-488-7386). In fact, take a moment to just put that in your phone right now—you never know when you or a friend may need it.

There are also a number of resources available for people dealing with (or wanting to help others deal with) minority stress and their effects:

- **The Association for Lesbian, Gay, Bisexual & Transgender Issues in Counseling** (algbtic.org) offers a list of resources for LGBT individuals and works to educate counseling professionals on GLBT issues.

- **The Association of Gay and Lesbian Psychiatrists** (aglp. org) offers numerous resources for LGBT people with mental health conditions, including a directory of GLBT-friendly therapists.

- **The LGBT National Help Center** (LGBThotline.org) provides multiple resources and access to a hotline (**888-843-4564**) and a youth chat line (**800-246-7743**).

- **The Pride Institute** (pride-institute.com) offers a GLBT residential treatment program, including psychiatric care for depression, anxiety, and other needs.

- **Trans Lifeline**, the first suicide hotline specifically for trans people (**877-565-8860**).

- **The Trevor Project** (TheTrevorProject.org) is a multimedia support network for LGBTQ youth providing crisis intervention and suicide prevention.

## CHAPTER TWENTY-NINE
# THE RELIGION THING

Religion is an important way that people identify themselves and make sense of their place in the world. Some religious beliefs and values might be in line with your sexual orientation or gender identity, and some may be in conflict.

Everyone has to navigate who they are spiritually with who they are physically, mentally, and emotionally. It is a very difficult thing for anyone to reconcile their biology and day-to-day choices with externally imposed moral sanctions, but many queer people do find a way to mesh their beliefs and identity together.

Children from all spiritual backgrounds including Buddhists, Christians, Jews, Muslims, and Sikhs can be bullied due to differences in their culture, traditions of dress, or specific beliefs.

People from all denominations have also used their religions to justify bullying others simply because they disapprove of their beliefs or perceived way of life. Much of this religious bullying is directed at GLBTQ people.

Religious bullying is particularly potent because it communicates an endorsement from a higher authority, suggesting that the hate has been sanctioned by adults, the governing, spiritual entity, and its representatives—making the impact feel bigger and more real than it actually is. Bullying of this nature, in churches, communities, schools, and at home, often goes beyond mere verbal and emotional abuse and can become physical as well.

LGBT youth targeted by religious bullying can feel so ostracized and unaccepted that they may make irrational decisions that hurt them later on such as leaving the church, dropping out of school, answering violence with more violence, or succumbing to (the sometimes suggested) suicide.

No one deserves to be bullied simply because they live or believe something different than someone else.

The problem is, there is a strong connection between religion and negative attitudes toward queer people.[1]

Much of the time, having a religious or philosophical dedication to something, a belief in something larger than ourselves and structured social, recreational, or religious activity, is associated with healthy and happy outcomes, like less depression and self-harm behaviors.[2]

However, GLBT people who grow up in toxic and (homo/bi/trans)-phobic environments, don't get the healthy and the happy parts—they get discrimination and confident-sounding messages that their creator and authority figures (who generally advocate for respect, tolerance, and good will) find them unacceptable, abominable, or even evil.

This can lead to negative thoughts and feelings directed at themselves because of who they are, who they love, or the body or gender to which they were born. This is called internalized homophobia or internalized transphobia.

Teenagers who experience these internalized phobias and/or discrimination from others due to their sexual orientation or gender identity have higher levels of suicidal ideation.[3]

Historically, many organized religions have treated LGBT people harshly. Despite some extremist, misguided, and hateful messages, it's very important to understand and believe that there is nothing inherently wrong with being GLBT. Now, within nearly every denomination there are supportive groups that have adopted healthier, more loving, welcoming, inclusive, and more-supportive stances toward the LGBT community.

As long as people are not injuring or impeding anyone else's life or liveliness, all people should be allowed to pursue their philosophies both religious and secular in peace.

If you find that you are being religiously bullied because of who you are or who you love, the following resources can be helpful.

- Pflag.org/Faith in Our Families

- Gaychurch.org

- ReligiousTolerance.org
- BelieveOutLoud.com (Christian GLBT support)
- IslamandHomosexuality.com (Muslim LGBT support)
- KeshetOnline.org (Jewish LGBT support)

## CHAPTER THIRTY
# IF YOUR FAMILY IS UNSUPPORTIVE . . .

I f your parents kick you out, it is not the end of the world (even though it may feel like it is). You can and will survive (even though you may feel like you won't).

It *will* get better.

Reach out to friends and extended family first—you will be surprised how caring people can be when they find that a parent has abandoned a child.

People do not have to become proper foster parents to help you, though if/when you find someone to take you in, and you are still legally a minor, you may want to contact your local child protective services. There is often a shortage of families willing or prepared to take in teens, so a family that elects to become a foster placement to take you in may not have much trouble becoming approved as foster parents. The financial support, benefits, and resources they can get as a foster parent may be helpful to both them and you.

If you don't have or can't find someone to stay with, and you are still legally a minor, you will want to contact your local child protective services anyway.

Be sure to tell them that you are LGBT and/or Q.

Also, contact the closest GLBT center (a state-by-state list can be found at **GayLife.About.Com**). They may be able to help steer you to a good foster home or LGBT-friendly group home.

If you are no longer a minor, you won't need child protective services, but I would still recommend contacting your local social services agency *and* your local GLBT center.

## Living on the Street

Do everything you can to avoid ending up living on the street. There is a long history of LGBTQ youth ending up as homeless, and for many that situation does not end well.

Living on the street can increase your level of desperation, need, and depression—all of which can lead to substance abuse. That can end you. Living in the street can lead to survival sex—trading sex acts for places to stay or food (or those drugs I just mentioned). Survival crime is a thing, too. Longtime activist and mentor Dan Savage famously says, It Gets Better, and I agree—unless you screw it up by racking up a long record of crimes and charges. This will impact how much people trust you and will damage your bigger reputation—plus jail time never looks good on a resume.

Too many teens end up badly through this route—trans, cis, gay, and straight, but approximately 40 percent of all American homeless youth identify as LGBTQ—most of whom have been disowned by someone.[1]

Because of that (grossly high) number, musician and longtime GLBTQ advocate Cyndi Lauper established the True Colors Fund (TrueColorsFund.org) and its Forty to None Network, which connects homeless LGBTQ youth to services and resources through a supportive, online community.

**If you are kicked out of your home:**

- Try to **take your ID, phone, and charger** with you!

- Reach out to a **friend or supportive family member**.

- Contact the **National Runaway Switchboard (800-621-4000)**.

- Speak to your **school counselor**.

- Call your local **Child Protective Services** agency.

- **211** is another great resource. Like calling 911 (for emergency services), calling 211 connects you to social services where referral specialists work with callers to assess their needs, determine their options, provide support and access to programs/services, and intervene in crisis situations.

- Contact your closest **LGBTQ resource center**—there is a state-by-state list on GayLife.about.com.

- Stay in / get back to **school**!

- Get a **job** as soon as possible.

- Explore **other resources** including HRC.org, NationalHomeless.org, and LambdaLegal.org.

- Specifically contact the **LGBT Youth Talkline,** a support hotline at **(800) 246-7743** (or email Help@LGBThotline.org).

The LGBT Youth Talkline provides (free and confidential) telephone, online private one-to-one chat, and email peer-support, as well as factual information and local resources for cities and towns across the United States.

Not just for when the poo hits the propeller, they claim the "Largest resource database" for GLBT youth in the world, with information on thousands of youth groups, social and support organizations, as well as queer-friendly religious organizations, sports leagues, and student groups.

**Above all:** hold onto yourself and make good choices. LGBTQ youth are abandoned and cast aside because someone believed that they were not worth holding onto. **Prove them wrong.**

## What If Your Family *Was* Unsupportive . . . But Now They Say They've Changed?

There may be situations in which some family members who were hurtful, unsupportive, or even cruel may gain some insight, learn new information, simply evolve as a person, or may not be able to deal with or heal from the void they created when they abandoned a queer person in their life.

Whether it's a parent, grandparent, sibling, or some other relational connection, if you have a family member who later finds you and wants to reconcile, here are some guidelines:

## Make Sure You Are Ready

Bounce the idea and plan off your friends, family, or even a therapist—it can be very tempting and even obligation-inducing to be contacted by an estranged family member—even one who has hurt you. People who care about you may be able to offer a more objective opinion about whether resuming contact is safe or smart.

Reconnection is easier if you have a solid base to stand on—such as a caring support system, a stable living situation, and some level of financial freedom.

You do not need to do anything you are not comfortable with or that may tempt you back into an unhealthy pattern, relationship, or living situation.

## Explore Their Motivations

Finding out why they want to meet with you is important to do *before* you actually meet. Sometimes their motivations will be honorable; they realized how wrong/hurtful they were, they genuinely feel sorry, or they have missed your presence in their life. If their motivations are more self-serving—such as making a good show for another family member, trying again to fix or save you, or to make themselves feel better—you do not have to engage.

## Tread Carefully

Like a latte that just burned you, that next taste should be small and cautious.

Meet in a public place that is either neutral or on your "turf" such as a restaurant, coffeehouse, park, or even a therapist's office. Ideally it should be a time and place that will not limit how long you can talk, but also where you can easily leave if you become uncomfortable.

Enlisting a friend or supportive other to be nearby or on call as an exit strategy or ride can help you feel confident and safe as well.

Under no circumstances do you need to work harder than they do to make a meeting happen. Even if they initiate the contact, you should be able to set the parameters—when, how long, and where you meet. If any travel is involved, it should be they who come to you.

## Consider What Information to Share

Ahead of time, you could write down or talk out with a friend or therapist what you want to say and how you want to say it. If you have anything to apologize for you can do that, but do not let them off the hook for doing the same.

You do not need to feel obligated to share with them any info about your work, home, school, friends, family, partner/s, or anything else about your day-to-day life. An initial meeting is about what has already happened, and you have plenty of time to think about what happens next—you do not need to rush into sharing access to your life with someone who hasn't yet earned it.

## Keep an Open Mind about What They Share

It is easy and understandable to have an idea or a hope about what they will do or say when you meet. Working to be open to the outcome, and not attached to things going down in a certain way, will protect your feelings and help you not be disappointed.

Let things happen naturally, and give both them and you time to say and process everything.

## Discuss Where To Go from Here

You may want to bring up what comes next before you leave (and, again, you may want to think this through ahead of time, so you don't feel pressured).

Even if the meeting goes well, apologies and forgivenesses are exchanged, and everyone has both cried and smiled, that does not mean that you necessarily want to continue to be in a relationship with them. It is OK if the meeting was simply a nice, successful one-time-thing.

If you think you are interested in ending the time you have spent without each other, you may want to set a time and place where you can meet with them again.

Healing will take time, for both you and them. So set another time and place to meet far enough in the future to give you time to process what has gone on, how the meeting went, and how you feel about going forward with the relationship.

## Reboot . . .

Every relationship is complicated—especially with family. *And* it is important to make an effort to start fresh after a reunification—being prepared to accept them where they are and expecting them to do the same for you.

None of you will be the same people you were last time you spoke, but what happens next is more important than what has already happened.

## . . . at Dial-Up Speed

It will be important for everyone involved to move slowly through this process. Jumping cannonball style back into old family patterns or flinging the door to your world wide open for them to come in could result in more tension, shock, and the same feelings and actions that caused the rift in the first place.

What happens next *is* more important than what has already happened, *and* the biggest predictor of future behavior is someone's past behavior. So, if there was *any* level of physical abuse directed at you or substance abuse that played into the problems before, it is a good idea to find out what steps they have taken to correct those things, such as anger management classes or recovery programs.

Your safety, both physical and emotional, is the most important thing here, and if they have not taken care of any secondary issues that played into how they treated you before, it is important to know that and to act accordingly.

## Keep Your Expectations Realistic and Your Boundaries Strong

There will be challenges, old arguments, hurt feelings, and new emotions, and that past you will be working to put behind you will pop up at times no matter what you do. Talk about these things as they happen.

Be clear with them what your expectations are if/when you move forward—such as using your chosen name, proper pronouns, or welcoming a partner to join you at Thanksgiving in their home.

Allow the new relationship to develop as slowly as it needs to, and give yourself (and them) opportunities to take a step back, make sure it is working, and respect that everyone needs to process their feelings (old and new) at their own pace.

# PART NINE

# "(SUPERMODEL) YOU BETTER WORK!"

Most of you reading this have probably thought of the Internet as a primary source of entertainment. At some point it is important to begin thinking of your technology differently, and taking it more seriously—as a tool, not simply a toy.

Online sites can range from educational to misleading, empowering to hateful, comedic to violent, and the lines dividing these things can be very fuzzy. Everyone interacting through the Web is going to encounter disturbing information, information that is racist, homophobic, sexist, and worse. As humans, it is hard to "unsee" things, which makes it very important to choose our media—particularly websites—very carefully.

Part of good digital citizenship is doing due diligence to avoid illegal content and other information that may promote hate speech, bigotry, or sexual or physical harm toward anyone based on their sex, gender, or orientation, or their race, nationality, language, age, or ability. Even if you have already begun streaming or downloading such content, it is never too late to pause, stop, or delete.

## CHAPTER THIRTY-ONE
# ONLINE SAFETY

The following information should not be given out online without a really good reason, proof of a secure and legitimate site, and your parents' permission if you are under the age of eighteen:

- your full name

- your parents' or siblings' full names

- your home address

- anyone's password/s

- phone numbers

- Social Security numbers

- credit card numbers

- the locations and schedules of your school, teams, or job.

When communicating with others through your screens, be particularly cautious when someone attempts to turn the chat to something other than the topic for which the app or site was designed, particularly if it is private information about yourself and especially if they are attempting to make the conversation sexual. Do not make physical contact with anyone you meet online without talking to a trusted adult first.

If you do decide to meet someone you only know online, make sure you

- meet in a public place (and stay there);

- verify their identification ahead of time, including a phone number they answer, or find their name and picture on a social networking site;

- give a parent or friend that information, or take someone with you.

According to the Crimes Against Children Research Center, one out of five US teenagers who are active online have received an unwanted sexual solicitation via the Internet.[1] These solicitations were sexual talk, requests to engage in sexual activities, or requests for personal information.

One-third of American teens have received an aggressive sexual solicitation in the past year.[2] This means a predator has

- asked a young person to meet somewhere,

- called a young person on the phone,

---

## LGBTW . . . IRL Dating

Online dating is a great way to meet interesting people, although in real life, it can also put you in potentially vulnerable situations with people you know nothing about, with no connection to coworkers, friends, or family.

It is super-important to remember that meeting someone in the real world that you have only met/known online can be dangerous—especially if you are underage. Always, always, let a responsible adult know before doing this, and meet in a public place.

Some people snap a picture of their date when they do meet, and text it to a friend (selfie-style) as a security measure. Anyone you choose to date who is mature, responsible, and cares about people's safety (in their life as well as in the larger community) will *not* be annoyed or offended by this. If they act put out or give you any level of crap for being appropriately cautious for your own safety, then don't let them date you.

---

- sent correspondence, money, or gifts through the US Postal Service.

Behaviors like these are called grooming. Grooming is a way that child molesters and other predators try to make people vulnerable, to drop their guard or get them to trust them. It can be hard to notice when people with bad intentions are trying to groom you, because grooming often feels good. Predators will give compliments, time, keep secrets, even give money, but in the end they will ask you to do something that is not smart, not safe, and probably sexual. Grooming is a flavor of manipulation, and groomed people often feel they owe the other person or are in some other way obligated to trust them or do what they say. Seventy-seven percent of the targets for online predators are fourteen and older, and 22 percent are ages ten to thirteen.[3]

The US Department of Justice maintains that, on average, there is one child molester per square mile in the United States.[4] Given isolated areas such as Kansas or the Appalachians and the vastness of places such as Texas and Alaska, this may not seem like such a big deal. However, if you acknowledge that the Internet transforms your computer screen into an open window between your home and virtually anyplace else in the world, these stats take on new meanings. Online gaming, social networking, and certain apps can make this job easier for predators.

The Breck Foundation (breckbednar.com) is a great online awareness resource for online safety and raising awareness about online grooming by predators.

If you or someone you know has been exploited, harassed, threatened, or groomed online

- tell your parents, a teacher or another concerned adult.

- notify your Internet service provider and/or the developer of the app, site, or game.

- call the CyberTipline online (cybertipline.com) or (800) 843-5678.

- call your local police.

# Human Trafficking

Human trafficking is when someone forces someone else to do labor and/ or sexual things in order to make money, such as forced prostitution, selling a kidnapped person as a "sex slave," or making someone pose for pornographic pictures. This kind of slavery happens all over the world. In fact, it is the third-largest international crime industry (right behind drugs and weapons trafficking).[5]

There are approximately ten million to thirty million slaves in the world today.[6] People of every race, age, religion, and gender can be trafficked, controlled, and forced to work or made to participate in the sex trade, though most of the human trafficking victims in the world are female-identified and younger than eighteen.[7]

Sex traffickers (often called "pimps") manipulate people (straight and gay) in person and online with promises of things like love, protection, escape, and adventure.

The average age of trafficked girls is about twelve to fourteen years old (boys are targeted a bit younger, at eleven to thirteen years old).[8] Some victims are targeted online and tricked into meeting someone pretending to be someone they are not; some are kidnapped forcefully; and some are even recruited by friends or classmates who have already been trafficked— many pimps use teens to recruit other young people.

Running away, being physically or sexually abused, having limited education or family support, and not being smart or safe online put teens at higher risk to be trafficked.

**To lower the risk of you or other people you know being trafficked:**

- Don't date people (particularly those who identify as men) who are out of high school and/or more than two years older than you—especially if you do not know them well, only know them online, or if they are going above and beyond their job description. It might feel like a compliment, but the older guy who wants to date someone in high school is either not mature enough to date people his own age, or is purposely seeking out younger people for some other, probably creepy reason. Think: once you are out of high school, are you planning to go back to high school to get dates?

- Date people your own age, and always make sure they are willing to meet your friends and family.

- Always trust your gut. Older people (men and women) who want you to model for pictures or be a client in their talent agency should always raise red flags. Be cautious, and if something seems weird or too good to be true, it probably is.

- Trust your friends' guts. If people you trust are giving you negative feedback about a relationship or situation, you should pay attention.

- Participate in activities that you enjoy and are good at. Confidence makes you less of a target.

- Don't share personal information on the Internet.

- Don't accept social media requests from unknown people. (Yes, even if they're hot.)

- Friend and follow your parents for safety reasons (and because you're a big kid).

- Don't share naked photos of yourself with your devices.

- Stop using the word *pimp* as a good thing. Pimps are criminals. They are violent; they abuse, control, and exploit people; and they steal money and lives that aren't theirs. This is not a compliment.

- Educate yourself about the issue of human trafficking at sites such as Polaris (polarisproject.org) and National Human Trafficking Resource Center (traffickingresourcecenter.org).

- Encourage your friends to do the same.

- Share your knowledge through links and posts on social media, and maybe even host an awareness event in your school or community.

- Say something if you see someone or something suspicious.

- In fact, **save (888) 373-7888 in your phone**. This is the twenty-four-hour hotline at the National Human Trafficking Resource

Center (texting "befree" to 233733 also connects you to the NHTRC). HumanTrafficking.org also provides information to combat trafficking through prevention, prosecution, and victim protection.

If you have concerns about trafficking for yourself or someone else:

- Tell a parent or another concerned adult.

- Call your local police.

- Call the National Human Trafficking Resource Center: (888) 373-7888 (or text "befree" to 233733).

# PORN

In the global village that is the World Wide Web, a plethora of information is available at our fingertips. This includes information and entertainment. Unfortunately, this also includes misinformation; racist, sexist, homophobic, transphobic, and other bigoted or violent information and images; and a ton of pornography.

According to a 2007 study from the University of Alberta, as many as 90 percent of boys and 70 percent of girls have been exposed to sexually explicit content at least once by the time they enter puberty.[1] This often happens accidentally, such as while completing their homework. Not only has porn moved from being an adult-only commodity, its quantity and intensity have both had their volumes turned way up, as it has seeped into almost every area of popular American culture.

There are very few kids who will not encounter pornography at some point by the time they begin high school, some during puberty,[2] and most certainly by the time they graduate from high school. Magazines that are legally restricted to adults are still kept behind those stupid plastic dividers in convenience stores and require ID for purchase, yet obscene, graphic, moving, high-definition images (of things that do not necessarily need to be in HD) are easily accessed online.

Several factors contribute to this, including

- the financial rewards for the producers who can make money from people's insecurities and natural inquisitiveness,

- the lack of a walled, online village for young people,

- the technology available to underagers and their knowledge of how to navigate it,

- the ease of posting and downloading amateur or homemade images and text as well as the pay-to-view stuff,

- unsolicited push porn, such as pop-up ads, banners, and key-word searches that turn even innocent and legitimate pages and searches into pathways to pornography exposure.

Porn, in particular, has a much different meaning than it did just a generation ago. Pornography used to be relatively hard to come by. In the 1980s, the average age of first exposure to pornography was sixteen. The average age of pornography exposure today is estimated to be eleven.[3] Young people today actually have to expend more energy to avoid pornography than their parents ever spent trying to get their hands on the stuff!

Porn can be particularly problematic for people who

- have not yet developed the ability (or even the motivation) to navigate relationships,

- have not had any education around sex or safety,

- are still impressionable and have yet to solidify their self-concepts,

- have bodies (as well as brains) that have not yet fully developed.

Porn objectifies women and men. It reduces them to parts and things, puts the first and primary focus on genitals, and eliminates any perceived need to connect with a partner emotionally or intellectually.

Porn can morph expectations around types and amounts of sex, stressing performance and conquest. It also deemphasizes safety measures and pacing, essentially hard-wiring a template that is only focused on one person's timing and needs.

Porn can perpetuate social awkwardness and anxiety. Many people do not grow into a confident sense of themselves until their twenties, but for those who rely on porn to feel satisfied and/or who use porn as an escape to avoid experiencing (the good and bad of) relationships, that time can be extended.

Porn sets impossible physical standards. Both males and females suffer from body issues associated with pornography consumption: the boy who doesn't have a ten-inch penis, the girl who isn't looking forward to having to bend in that position or be called that name, the guy who doesn't have that six-pack, the girl who doesn't have that thigh gap, the kid who maybe doesn't want sex at every given moment of any given day, the kid who has found that shaving their genitals is actually itchy and super uncomfortable. . . .

The larger culture of the porn industry itself can contribute sometimes to bigger-picture issues such as mistreatment of the actors, misogyny, and encouraging rape culture.

But porn is not inherently or completely negative or unhealthy in and of itself; rather like shopping, video games, or french fries, it is one's relationship to the porn that determines how healthy (or not) it is.

The younger the porn consumer, the more vivid and impactful those problems become.

Incorporating pornography into an already established sexual lifestyle or sense of yourself as a sexual person is *very* different than creating those things out of pornography.

Adult use can help people discover what pleases them sexually, expose them to new ideas, and provide validation of thoughts and feelings, but consuming graphic, moving, HD images of unrealistic bodies doing unrealistic things as an adolescent can have negative impacts on developing psyches, minds, and attitudes.

The reality is that most people's brains and personalities aren't quite done "cooking" until around their twenties. And if your coming out was a struggle or a challenge, or if you have discovered and begun a completely new invention of yourself through transition, this period could be extended even to age twenty-five. This writer recommends abstinence for your developing brain, developing self-concept and developing libido, and understanding exactly how porn can have an impact on your expectations about sex, sexuality, and relationships.

People can tell, for example, if someone has learned how to "do sex" by watching porn. And they do not typically consider it a good thing.

Whether or not you wait until adulthood to consume porn, it is wise to create limits around it (again, just like french fries).

One good rule of thumb is to not let it take up more than 50 percent of the time you masturbate. For the other 50 percent, masturbate using only your brain and imagination. This is important because relying only on screens means you use zero imagination while jacking/jilling off or when in a sexual situation with a partner. Imagination is crucial for flirting, dating, and maintaining things such as empathy and romance in real relationships.

More than just paying attention to how much porn you choose to use, going at porn like a grown-up involves being choosey about what porn you watch as well. Limiting your viewing to only authentic brands on tube sites, streaming rather than downloading, and exploring feminist porn (which focuses on more balanced acts that give everyone pleasure) can help you be more ethical, more aware of the ages and working conditions of actors, and avoid viruses and other questionable content.

There is some good news, in terms of the differences between typical, mainstream straight porn and typical, mainstream gay porn.

In gay porn:

- **Body hair** is more prevalent—typically one has to search specifically for a lack of body hair. In straight porn, body hair—including pubic hair—is almost nonexistent.

- There is more **reciprocity** in terms of power dynamics and behavior.

- **Non-sexual affection** is more often displayed—including hugging, kissing, and even flirting.

- **Condoms are the typical default**. One has to specifically search for non-condom ("bareback") sex.

- There is a **wider/more realistic range in body types**.

That being said, there are still cautions. You are watching too much porn if you are

- watching porn every single, bloody day;

- choosing porn instead of spending time with people;

- having problems in your life because of porn, such as getting into trouble at home, school, or work, overspending, getting computer viruses, or upsetting people you care about;

- can't or won't stop even after those consequences;

- are looking at more porn than you used to have to;

- are looking at things in porn that would be illegal in real life (like anything involving animals or little kids);

- are "porn-ifying" your day-to-day life—thinking about what he would look like naked, or if she would do that thing from that video—or if you find yourself sexualizing fantasy and animated characters;

- not liking yourself because you don't date porn stars, because you still have all of your pubic hair, or because your body parts aren't as big as those actors';

- feeling rejected, inadequate, and unable to compete;

- feeling guilty for telling your partners they are being too rough, demanding, or rude during sex;

- having trouble getting aroused, hard, or wet unless you are viewing images.

It is important to remember that porn is not real—it is sexual, but it is not about sex. It is important to make sure that you do not let porn use warp your values, your self-esteem, or your sense of self as a sexual person. It is important to keep in mind that, though it may take more effort, emotional risk, and energy, IRL interactions and relationships are far more rewarding than anything you can experience alone with a screen.

## CHAPTER THIRTY-THREE
# DIGITAL CITIZENSHIP

Digital citizenship refers to the cultural rules and customs of appropriate, mannerly, responsible, and safe behavior online and through our screens. Self-care, self-concept, and relationships also extend to our technological lives, including how we interact with others, flirting, and keeping our antennae (and speakers) tuned for dangers. **Social networking** allows you to

- stay connected with friends and family.

- meet and interact with others who share similar interests.

- get involved with groups, clubs, or teams.

- up your creativity through the sharing of ideas, music, and art.

- provide an emotional support network.

- show the world how awesome you are.

And then there is the abyss, which everyone is tempted to fall into from time to time. It is important to make sure you balance your screen time with real, human interaction and physical activities. Online interaction is meant to pass the time—not fill it.

The American Academy of Pediatrics recommends that teens spend no more than ten to fifteen hours a week engaged in entertainment media. That works out to an hour or two per day.[1] You should not be using online entertainment more than you are doing your homework or spending time with other humans in real life. Online interaction is meant to be an adjunct or a cool addition to warm, human contact—not a replacement. Allowing your social networking to be the primary focus of your time, energy, or relationships can increase attention issues, lower your general, physical health, cause sleep and school problems, and atrophy your in-real-life means and muscles of making friends and getting dates. Don't do this.

Just like real life, social networking comes with its own set of rules and ways to behave.

The following guidelines can help you protect your reputation, your loved ones, and yourself as you interact through your screens[2]:

**No one is ever as anonymous as they think they are, and what you post today can come back to haunt you later. The Internet is Forever.**

- Use privacy settings and options for limiting messages, and manage your updates and audiences to increase your freedom to be your authentic self online.

- Set regular dates to review and update your privacy policies.

- Do not speak negatively on your feed about friends, enemies, exes, parents, teachers, or bosses.

- Avoid constant negativity, cussing, oversharing, spoiling, poor grammar, and misspellings.

- Remember that, much like a tattoo, the nudity, grotesque or funny jokes, *Jackass*-style antics, or explicit song lyrics you post today will still be associated with you in the future.

- Remember that your future in-laws, employers, college registrars, and grandchildren will likely be able to see your posts.

- Check the facts of your updates and sources of your news before posting so you don't look like an idiot. (Snopes.com is your friend.)

- Friend and follow only people you want to be associated with. Don't be shy about unfriending people you no longer feel comfortable being connected to or associated with.

- Likewise, don't be shy about untagging yourself from photos or asking others to remove photos of you from their pages if such posts jeopardize your comfort, relationships, or reputation.

- Do not tag others in photos or posts without permission, especially if they include risky or embarrassing behavior.

- When other people express hate and complain, strive to ignore rather than engage with them.

- Do not waste time or energy trying to correct those people who use social networking to spread hate or lies.

- Do not post when rushing, exhausted, drunk, high, driving, or really, really pissed off.

**Remember that social networking accompanies real-world interaction, and that it does not replace it.**

- Balance your online life with real, warm human contact; socially responsible, and age-appropriate activities; relationships; and physical exercise.

- Realize that friending online is not the same as real life, and that the number of friends you have online is not a real-world badge of how cool, popular, interesting, or hot you are.

- Unplug from technology when in the company of family, friends, colleagues, and clients.

- Don't allow social networking to replace the "realness" of face-to-face communication.

- Remember that it's social media, not your diary or therapist.

- Don't make it easier for strangers to connect with you more than your own loved ones.

**Understand that to err is human, but to seriously aggravate a situation requires an Internet connection.**

- Do not share passwords with anyone except your parents.

- Be respectful of the rules and always follow the terms of use for the social platform you are using.

- Spellcheck is your friend.

- While you're at it, actually spell out words.

- Do not post anything you wouldn't say in a face-to-face interaction.

- Actual human beings read the words you post, text, or send, so remember, your computer does not give you free rein to be cruel or rude.

- Have a litmus test for whom you friend or follow. For example, only people you would invite to your house for dinner or buy a birthday gift for.

**Understand that while you are online, manners still matter. Tweet others the way you want to be tweeted.**

- Remember that kindergarten rules such as saying "please" and "thank you" still apply.

- Show patience and kindness to newbies.

- Do your legitimate best to not offend anyone with your content.

- Do not tweet or post from the bathroom.

- Be mindful about what personal information you share, but use your real picture, real name, and real age in your profile.

- Choose a picture that reflects how you would like to be perceived by your friends, family, and associates.

- Don't spoil it when you live-tweet sporting events, award ceremonies, elections, or season finales. Post spoiler alerts, so people can take a break from your feed for the night. Otherwise, wait a day or two before posting specific spoilers.

- Speaking of spoiling, do not "vulture" other people's posts by posting about others getting married, pregnant, or raises; moving; breaking up; or coming out until they post it first.

- Do not call out, humiliate, or gossip about people online—it's social networking, not reality television.

- Do not poach others' friend lists just because you think someone is hot. Ask for an introduction first.

- When you send friend requests to people you do not know well, attach a message with an introduction.

- Beware of oversharing and avoid topics such as bodily functions, anything involving bodily fluids, and personal hygiene mishaps.

- Balance your feeds with philosophical and funny, positive and negative, the silly and the cerebral.

- Give love by being charitable with other people's observations and content, and don't just talk about yourself.

---

## LGBTW . . . Apps

There are loads of apps out there that encourage sneaky, inappropriate, and sometimes illegal behavior. It is important, in the service of being a responsible person, to not spend your time, energy, or money investing in apps that

- mask your identity,

- promote cruel behavior,

- encourage you to lie,

- help you break the law, or

- make it easy to be located by people you do not know.

Using those apps gives your time, energy, and money to developers who encourage irresponsible behavior, take advantage of stupid people, and support the predators who prey on them.

---

**Sexting** is generally defined as sending sexually graphic images, videos, and text messages over media lines.

Though adults do this, it is a different situation when it involves minors, and this trend of sending sexual texts and pictures via cell phones has led to a number of teens being charged with child pornography.[3]

## Things to Know About Digital Flirting

Since the beginning of time, everyone in every generation has done something out of character, something impulsive, something stupid, something dangerous, maybe even illegal. The thing is, throughout the ages, unless that thing got you arrested, killed, or did the same to someone else, you generally enjoyed the luxury of working it out of your system and having the event fade quietly into forgotten history and riding off into the metaphorical sunset.

Now, however, technology is within an arm's reach of everyone and our every move, scandalous and sublime, sweet and sucky, gets posted and passed to our friends and their friends and their friends. Nothing gets worked out anymore, there is no forgetting, and that sunset has been replaced by The Cloud. The Internet is Forever.

And you will be twenty someday, and thirty-five, and hopefully sixty. You will have job interviews, and possibly in-laws. College registrars and your own, potential grandchildren are going to be able to Google your ass.

So when flirting digitally, keep it PG-13; stick to compliments, questions, and comments about things that have already happened. Keep your

---

### LGBTW . . . Child Pornography[4]

Any naked image of anyone younger than eighteen can be defined as child pornography—even if it is their own bits and pieces.

It is a felony to create child pornography.
It is a felony to distribute child pornography over media lines.
It is a felony to possess child pornography.
Felony. Felony. Felony.

Under federal law, child pornography is a criminal act, and is defined as any kind of drawing, cartoon, sculpture, painting, photograph, film, video, computer-generated image, or picture that depicts a minor engaging in obscene, sexually explicit conduct.[5] These illegal images can be produced and presented in various forms, including print media, videotape, film, CD, the Internet, and yes, cell phones, and teens found distributing or possessing such images can be found guilty of child pornography.

In fact, it is only called "sexting" when *everyone* involved is older than eighteen. Otherwise, it's child pornography.

Any sexualized picture or text you create, send, or pass on could end up blasted out by someone else to people (and numbers of people) that you do not want, could be traced back to you bringing (personal, legal, and safety) consequences with them and could potentially find their way into the bigger-picture, supply-and-demand culture of online child pornography.

---

clothes on, listen to your gut, and trust your instincts. If something tells you it is not the right time or person, do not hit "send."

I want to challenge each of you reading this to care enough about yourself to choose the attention you get from your suitors (male or female, straight or gay, trans or cis) on purpose. This means:

- Move at your own pace, and demand they first give attention to the beauty and fantastic things you have to offer under your skin, not just under your clothes.

- Make them appreciate what's between your ears more than what's between your legs.

- Wait for them to show interest and curiosity about your heart before you let them anywhere near your crotch.

## Cyberbullying

Cyberbullying is when someone embarrasses, harasses, threatens, or attacks someone else by using technology, such as phones, computers, and tablets, as well as social media sites, text messages, chat, apps, and websites.[6]

Examples of cyberbullying include

- forwarding personal or private messages or pictures;

- posting pictures without consent;

- writing mean, scary, or violent text messages, posts, or emails;

- spreading rumors or lies by email, text, or social media posts;

- posting embarrassing pictures, videos, or memes;

- using fake pages, memes, or profiles;

- using modifying software to publicly embarrass someone with fake pictures or memes;

- catfishing/tricking other people online into saying or doing things that are vulnerable or embarrassing;

- making direct threats or personal attacks; and

- "subtweeting"—spreading rumors, lies, or mean comments on any platform (not just Twitter) about someone without naming them directly, but using enough information so that everyone (usually including the victim) knows who is being discussed. It still counts as cyberbullying.

Mean comments and damaging rumors are the most common types of cyberbullying. Revenge, justice, and "just 'cuz" are the most common reasons given for it. Social networking sites and texts are the most common vehicles.

The psychological and emotional effects of cyberbullying are similar to those of real-life bullying, but can be much more damaging.

- In real life, bullying often ends when the school day ends, but cyberbullying can happen twenty-four hours a day, seven days a week. This means that people can still be bullied and humiliated even in their own homes.

- Mean and embarrassing information can be posted anonymously and distributed quickly to a very wide audience. This embarrassment feels large and public, and it often is.

- Deleting, stopping, or refuting the harassment or rumors is extremely difficult after the messages, texts, or pictures have been posted or sent.

- Unlike bullying that occurs in person, there are not usually teachers or other adults available to offer intervention, protection, or help and support, so victims often are left feeling very alone.

## Things to Understand About Cyberbullying

The anonymity that screens enable is very tempting, even for adults—just witness the comment threads underneath any given online article, the seemingly endless clickbait articles online ("12 childhood actors who grew up looking horrible!") that if they happened at your high school would result in suspensions. Even the online behavior of some high-ranking politicians is shockingly cruel and purposely timed and designed to harm other people.

Male-identified people tend to be more aggressive when they bully each other; female-identified people do more damage to each other through more passive or subtler ways, such as relational bullying.

Relational bullying can look like this:

- spreading rumors or gossip from the bully,

- sending or forwarding messages for or from the bully,

- encouraging the bully by laughing or liking their behavior or posts, or

- standing by and saying or doing nothing.

Everyone who interacts with other humans on the Internet witnesses cruel behavior, and anyone can become a target—in fact, almost half of all teens say they have been bullied online.[7] Even if you haven't been a direct victim of it, you likely know someone who has.

This particular kind of violence can be "contagious" in a way. Sixty-six percent of teens who have witnessed online cruelty have also witnessed others joining in.[8] Thirty-four percent of those who have had any engagement in cyberbullying have been both a cyberbully and been cyberbullied.[9]

Some people do not understand the consequences their behavior can have on the other end of a media line, some do not care, and others cross lines by accident. Thoughtless and irresponsible posting can be just as damaging as active bullying. Interactions through screens lack a large amount of what makes up human communication:

- eye contact;

- body language;

- tone of voice;

- facial expressions;

- physical emblems ("signs" that replace words, like a thumbs up or the middle finger);

- regulators (sounds that we use to give feedback, like "uh-huh" or "yum");

- adaptors (unconscious physical feedback clues like yawning when bored or biting your nails when nervous);

- proxemics (how we use space when communicating like taking a step back or leaning forward); and

- para language (emphasizing certain words as with sarcasm).

The above are all generally missing in online communications, and what little strategically placed punctuation and emojis make up for, the rest can contribute to accidental harm and hurt feelings for other people.

So, pay attention to not only how others treat you online, but how you treat others, and if you hurt someone in an online interaction, apologize and make it right, because cyberbullying can cause depression, feelings of isolation, and low self-esteem. There are many other negative effects, but these particular three also happen to be three major risk factors for suicide among teens.[10] Cyberbullying can escalate extremely quickly, and the consequences can be tragic. Studies show that 10 percent of cyberbullying victims contemplate suicide—three times more than kids who are not cyberbullied.[11]

## What To Do About Cyberbullying

If you witness anyone being bullied online, do not just stand by. You can help support the victim (as well as future victims) by standing up for a friend and telling a trusted adult, such as a teacher, parent, or coach. Save the posts to show as evidence. Above all, do not fight bullies by becoming one.

## What To Say to Someone Who Has (or You Think Might Have) Been Bullied

- Tell them what you heard.

- Ask if they are OK.

- Tell them it is not their fault.

- Let them know you do not agree with what happened.

- Tell them not to reciprocate.

- Encourage them to tell an adult.

- Offer to help them do that.

- Offer to do something social with them, lunch, studying, an activity after school, etc.

- Let them know you are there for them.

- Check in with them later.

## What Else Can You Do?

- Remember that bullies, at their core, are victims, too. They are not more powerful than you. That's why they are doing this so publicly—they are trying to make you *think* they are more powerful.

- Remember that by crossing the line, breaking school rules or sometimes the law by bullying you, bullies give all of their power up to you.

- Use your words, not your device. Tell someone, so the bully can be caught and punished.

- Then, use your device and block their ass.

- It is important to never, ever respond to a cyberbully; that only makes it worse. If you want to show someone you are upset, show your friends and family, who will support you. Showing the bullies you are upset will encourage them to continue targeting you.

- Do not lash out if you have been victimized. Seek help.

- If your school does not have a policy about cyberbullying, call school administrators on it, or get your parents to do it.

- Mind your friend lists and privacy settings.

- Create strong passwords, and never, ever give them out (even to your closest friend).

- Do not let someone use your phone or take your place at the computer and pretend to be you.

- Educate yourself and others about the effects of cyberbullying.

- Do not stay silent when someone else is harassed online. Report violent, sexual, and hateful behaviors to school administrators, parents, and/or police when necessary.

# PART TEN

# "WE ARE FAMILY"
# (FOR PARENTS)

Nearly every parent of a queer child has known on some level that their child was "different." That child has often known too. Once you've gotten to the point at which your child's "queerness" can be talked about between you, you will each feel fear, apprehension, awkwardness, and other flavors of angst—but there will also be relief, solace, and a sense of bonding between you as well.

But did you think the hard part was over?

When a queer kid comes out to their parents, the parent-child dynamic shifts, just as it can when school starts, puberty hits, or they move out on their own. Processing your child's definitive statement of their alternative sexuality or gender is only the beginning of your journey as a parent. You've freaked out a little (or were totally fine with it), you accept it, you support them—now you still have to parent them. . . .

## CHAPTER THIRTY-FOUR
# WHY THIS BOOK IS NECESSARY

The daily stress that comes with existence for GLBTQ adolescents cannot be ignored.

Lesbian, gay, bisexual, and trans adolescents follow developmental pathways that are both similar to and different from those of heterosexual/cisgender adolescents. All teenagers face certain developmental challenges, such as developing social skills, thinking about career choices, and fitting into a peer group. *But* what can feel normative for straight/cis youth can feel more challenging, even more political, for LGBT youth.

Social or political agendas or programs—including and especially at schools—that encourage prejudice against LGBT youth or that fail to create a welcoming and safe space for them, contribute to a wide range of negative outcomes for these young people including:

- lack of sex/prevention education

- disclusion/invisibility

- negative impacts regarding health

- violence

For example:

Despite the nearly one million queer teenagers in the United States,[1] and the growing acceptance of gays and lesbians in American popular culture, gay and lesbian teens are particularly uninformed and alienated by sex education classes.

American sex education standards vary widely across the country, though what many of them have in common is that they leave many American youth uninformed about the range of sex and sexuality—in everything from basic anatomy and relationship standards to safer sex and certainly sexual and gender diversity.

The majority of mainstream, school-based, sex education programs do not regularly or reliably talk about sexual orientation or gender identity. Some of this exclusion is on purpose, and some of it is because of ignorance. Worse still, for some programs that do include orientation and gender in the conversation, the information can be inaccurate—even negative.

Typical sex education often assumes students are heterosexual and cisgender. Many sex education curricula do not even mention sexual orientation or gender identity, and some others only describe it in a negative light if/when they do.

We are trembling on the edge of a turning point in history. At the time of this writing, only twelve states require discussion of sexual orientation in sex education, and, of those, four require the teaching of inaccurate and negative information (yeah, Alabama, South Carolina, Texas, and Utah—I'm looking at you). Some states take this even further, making explicitly negative statements about GLBT people and their relationships (hello, Arizona and Oklahoma). Only four US states currently mandate discussion of gender identity in sex education at all.[2,3]

Painting LGBT issues in this way implies that the youth these discussions benefit are, themselves, unacceptable, not worthy of inclusion, or unnatural. One day, the people in charge of and supporting these decisions (and their grandchildren) are going to look back on these choices and cringe, but right now, this is the reality we are dealing with.

Most school districts in this country advocate some form of sex education, but very few include resources and education for lesbians and gays in their curriculum. In fact, the only sex that is often discussed (and which kids are encouraged to abstain from) is penis-in-vagina intercourse.

When unethical and incomplete sex education curricula assume and assert heterosexuality as the norm, GLBT youth are left clueless about health and relationship dynamics, and are often forced to default to the Internet for the answers and information and community they seek.

Without the opportunity to be educated about the subject, some teens conclude that oral and anal sex are not real sex and therefore must not have the same risks or consequences. In fact, it is often referred to without the word *sex* included, as in "getting oral" or "we did anal last night."

In addition to fueling dangerous ignorance and contributing to hostile home, spiritual, and school environments, this thinking is also a significant risk factor for HIV and other sexually transmitted infections. It is critical that we open the lines of communication and help queer youth protect their sexual health, because queer youth are impacted more negatively than non-queer youth in terms of health issues.

Younger men (thirteen to twenty-nine) who have sex with other men make up two-thirds of new HIV infections.[4] The Centers for Disease Control and Prevention also report that men who have sex with men also account for about two-thirds of new syphilis cases.[5]

Yes, syphilis is still a thing (see chapter 20).

High school girls who identify as LG or B are more likely to contract an STI and/or become pregnant than their straight counterparts.[6] Transgender (and other gender nonconforming) youth experience higher rates of sexual assault.[7] And among trans youth, HIV rates are more than four times the national average.[8]

LGBT students who experience frequent harassment at school report lower grade-point averages than those who are not.[9]

Stigma and discrimination in school also lead to disproportionately high rates of mental-health issues among queer kids.[10]

In what is called the minority stress effect (see chapter 28), GLBT youth, like other oppressed minorities, may turn to substance use and other risk behaviors to cope with the stress of stigma and discrimination, resulting in self-esteem and higher rates of anxiety and depression and suicide. In addition to suicide, these kids are at increased risk for pregnancy and disease (as queer kids are less likely than their straight counterparts to prepare for sexual encounters).

LGBT people face higher rates of violence both at home and school than any other minority group, as well.[11] In fact, lesbian, gay, bisexual, and transgender people are the most likely targets of hate crimes in America, according to the Federal Bureau of Investigation.[12]

In the National Coalition of Anti-Violence Programs' (NCAVP) 2016 annual report outlining hate-driven violence,[13] they found the most common types of hate-based violence directed at GLBT people were verbal harassment (15 percent), discrimination (14 percent), physical violence (12 percent), and threats or intimidation (11 percent). Thirty-eight percent of the targets were youth and young adults.

Ironically, part of the reason for this violence has to do with the growing acceptance of queerness over the last few decades. As society as a whole becomes more exposed and tolerant of LGBT minorities, those who are opposed to the shift in culture become more activated—sometimes in extreme and violent ways. LGBTQ homicide rose 20 percent between 2014 and 2015.[14]

What makes this the most troubling is that queer kids are four times as likely as their straight counterparts to attempt suicide, according to the American Journal of Public Health.[15] More than half of transgender and gender nonconforming youth who experience harassment, assault, or discrimination in school attempt suicide.[16] Recent national studies indicate that suicide is the leading cause of death for lesbian, gay, bisexual, transgender, and questioning (LGBTQ) youth.[17]

What this means is that even the people who survive and move past or through fear, hatred, and violence directed at them for others are *still* at risk for "aftershock" harm—learning to direct that fear, hatred, and violence at themselves.

More and more evidence-based studies indicate that positive discussion of GLBT people, history, and issues in schools, media, and popular culture helps build safer environments in society in general, and decreases the educational, mental, and physical harms that LGBT youth experience, overall.

It is important to create safe environments for young people, whether they are straight, cis, L, G, B, or T. All youth thrive when they feel intellectually empowered, socially accepted, and emotionally and physically supported and safe.

This starts at home.

## Parents who are supportive of their LGBTQ child/ren:

- Provide safety, supervision, and support in their home.

- Do not define their child/ren by their sexuality.

- Model sexually healthy attitudes in their own relationships.

- Exhibit an open/non-shaming stance toward sexuality and gender.

- Exhibit a balanced/fair stance toward sexuality and gender.

- Are knowledgeable about sexuality and gender.

- Are knowledgeable about sexualities and genders different than their own.

- Discuss sexuality and gender with their child/ren.

- Take their child's coming out seriously, not assuming that, because they are young, they don't understand themselves or their sexuality.

- Ask their child/ren questions.

- Remain consistent with regard to affection, activities, conversation, and limits after they come out/transition.

- Seek and create opportunities to discuss sexuality with their child/ren.

- Demonstrate respect, boundaries, acceptance, and understanding, and trust in their child/ren.

- Utilize resources around sexuality.

- Prioritize their child's health, fulfillment, and happiness over traditional ideas of relationships, and rites of passage.

- Know that this is hard to do, and are gentle and compassionate with themselves.

- Share their sexual values with their child/ren and help them develop their own.

- Stay calm in the face of differing values and changing development.

- Maintain a solid stance around concepts such as equality, consent, and safety.

- Set and maintain limits for dating and other activities outside of the home.

- Regularly and overtly offer themselves as a support and a resource.

- Do not take offense when their child/ren do not wish to see them as such.

- Provide access to additional/optional support and resources— including health care.

- Do not indulge in stereotypes about gay/trans people.

- Find ways to connect and stay actively involved in the child/ren's lives.

- Find ways to connect and stay actively involved in their child/ren's lives—especially as they begin developing and dating.

- Feel pride and honor that their child has chosen to be honest and shared something deeply personal about themselves.

- Act accordingly.

# LGBTQ 101 FOR PARENTS

Transgender and gay/lesbian/bisexual people, issues, and culture have overlap, but gender identity is *not* the same as sexual orientation.

Sexual orientation describes a person's feelings of attraction toward same- or opposite-sexed people in relationship to their own.

Being trans (or cis) gender is about a person's internal sense of gender identity—the ways that people act, interact, or feel about themselves, which are associated with boys/men and girls/women.

Everyone possesses both a gender identity and a sexual orientation; in other words, a transgender person can also identify as gay, lesbian, or bisexual. . . .

And while children who eventually come out as lesbian, gay, or bisexual express gender atypical behaviors when younger, whether they are transgender is about identity rather than attraction.

Being transgender (or somewhere on that spectrum with cisgender) is about one's gender identity, while being gay (or somewhere on that spectrum with straight) is about one's sexual orientation.

Just as a cisgender man can be straight or gay, or a cisgender woman can be lesbian or straight, trans persons can be in different places on that spectrum as well. For example, a man who was gendered as a female at birth, but who later identifies as a man, can also be gay or straight (or anywhere on that spectrum). Identifying (genderly) as trans does not necessarily mean one must identify alternatively sexually as well. This can be hard to wrap your brain around, especially in situations in which (for example) a natal woman, identifying as female, might be attracted to and date women—identifying as lesbian or bi while doing so. That same person may later transition to a man and find himself still attracted to women—but identifying as straight (and trans). In fact most trans people find that, after they transition, they are attracted to the same gender they were prior to transition.[1]

Sexuality is a complicated dynamic that is not just about genetics and genitals—it's an ongoing and dynamic process that is influenced by genes, experience, family, personality, hormones, and environment, and some people do not develop a clear understanding of their sexual orientation or their gender identity until their teens or adulthood. Lack of inclusion, knowledge, and awareness can also contribute to this, as do fear, rejection, active prejudice, and violence.

Despite these things, many other LGB and T people developed an awareness of being LGB or T as soon as they knew what "boys" and "girls" were.

What awareness and coming out looks like can be different for each person—what matters is that they are supported as they sort it out.

Children are not born knowing what it means to be a boy or a girl. Children are typically set on a social and cultural trajectory as soon as they are born and their external sex organs are observed. As children pubesce, adult expectations of masculine and feminine expression and behavior often become encouraged and enforced by parents, their larger community, and media.

But we now know that gender does not simply exist in a polarized way; either "boy" or "girl"—it is a spectrum in which most everyone with human parts expresses and identifies with different aspects of both masculinity and femininity.

All children will engage in behaviors (stereotypically) associated with both boys and girls—some will play with trucks, some with dolls, or they may learn to cook or play guitar. Some will refuse to dress up or to associate with a particular color. Some will insist on singing showtunes or cuddling with stuffed animals.

Expectations of "What Girls Do" and "What Boys Do" have changed in the last few decades. All children show some behaviors that were once thought of as typical for the opposite gender. With evolutions in culture and technology, no one shows exclusively male or female traits anymore. Not even grown-ups.

That being said, there *are* societally prescribed boundaries around gender and behavior based on time, geography, and culture.

When a child's interests and abilities are different than those expectations, they are often subjected to discrimination and bullying. Sometimes as part of that bullying, and sometimes to help their child avoid said bullying, some parents become overly concerned with whether their child's interests and strengths coincide with socially defined gender roles of the moment/place/family/and so on, and spend unnecessary (and sometimes harmful) energy to mold (or force) their child's behavior into more traditional gender behavior.

Children need to feel comfortable with and good about themselves. Each child has his own strengths, which may or may not conform to society's (or your own cultural) expectations. When encouraged, those behaviors become a source of their current and future self-esteem, identity, and success.

Gender nonconforming behavior is developmentally normative, and behavior that is culturally different than the gender a child was assigned at birth does not necessarily mean that a child is gay, lesbian, or transgender.

Except when it does.

## CHAPTER THIRTY-SIX
# IS MY KID GAY?

C hildren are sexual creatures and can exhibit sexual behaviors throughout childhood. Even before birth, some babies have erections while still in the uterus, and some are born with an erection. Little boys and girls can experience orgasm from rubbing their genitals. As they get older they are curious and mimic adult behavior they see at home, in public, and in the media.

This may make some parents cringe (we don't like to think of them as sexual creatures any more than they appreciate thinking of us that way), but sexual curiosity and behavior is universal, normative, and, though it can involve gender atypical behavior and/ or same sex peers at times, is not an indication of future, sexual orientation.

Once puberty hits, children's curiosity and play become more activated and can become more distinctly sexualized—where they used to play "house" or "doctor," they may now play "Spin-The-Bottle," "Truth-Or-Dare," or social media versions of those same, intriguing dynamics.

The general rule is: the more developed their body is, the more curious and interested they become, and by pubescence, most children begin figuring out who they are attracted to sexually.

Whether and when and with whom they actually do anything sexual depends on a host of factors, including social, environmental, and biological factors. Though they may or may not be developed, may or may not be active, and may or may not be gay, sometime between the ages of nine and twelve is a good time to find resources for yourself, get informed, and begin having a conversation with your child about sexuality, sexual behavior, and sexual orientation.

Finding ways to inquire about your child's experience, offering yourself (and other sources) as a means to reliable information, and accepting your child (gay, straight, or anywhere in between) will help keep them safe as they mature.

There is no test or scanning system that can identify LGBT people. If your kid is queer, they are queer and have been since the day you first brought them home—whether you knew it at the time or not.

Parents and parenting do not make kids gay (and cannot turn them straight), but parents and parenting can make a child either happy or miserable. The reality is that most of us will do both throughout our parenting career, but if you think that your child might be some flavor of not-straight, here are some tips to create a safe space in your home.

## Tips for Parents of LGBTQ Children

### Understand that your child might be queer.

They are made of human parts, and some humans beings are gay, some are not. Some humans are cis, some are not. It's just science and probability . . .

### Use media.

Politics, song lyrics, commercials, and television and movie plots can all spark conversation around gay issues and dynamics, allowing you to voice support and concern in a casual way as well as acknowledging that you know there are all kinds of people and families in the world.

### Make your house more queer friendly.

Having books by or about queer people on the shelf, supportive stickers on the fridge, articles on the coffee table, or having your family participate in walks, rallies, and fund-raising for queer causes and rights sends a very clear, positive message.

### Let your kid be different.

Whether your kid is gay or straight, you may have a son who enjoys playing with dolls or redecorating the living room or a daughter who spends time working on the car or playing baseball. What parent hasn't had to sit through mind-numbing children's television programming or listened to how those remarkably and deeply complicated collectible card games work? Supporting your child's interests—even if it makes you uncomfortable—is showing your child that you respect them.

## Behave as though there were a queer person in the room.

Not telling or laughing at gay jokes, not using demeaning terms or slights about gay people or things, using open-ended language and questions, and learning terms *not* to say. Along the same lines, do not put up with hate speech from others—in the grocery store, in church, at the family picnic—silence in the face of overt anti-queer rhetoric implies consent—and your kid *will* notice. Clean up your messes if you've left a trail of unhelpful comments, terms, or jokes that you now realize were offensive or degrading.

## Remember that they are a minority—even if you are not.

Most minorities are based on race and/or religion—things that tend to run generationally in families. But most parents of queer kids are straight. In minority families, being a minority is a more natural and seamless part of the family structure and everyday dynamics; the politics and history are discussed, and traditions and rituals are passed down through generations. *You* may not be GLBT, but it is now your job to become an expert in this minority. Learn LGBT history, talk about the politics, create the traditions. . . .

## Ask them.

It can be OK to simply ask your child if they are gay or lesbian or bisexual or how they identify sexually. Even the most well-intentioned parent risks possibly traumatizing the kid who isn't (or isn't ready, or isn't comfortable), if you haven't done the prerequisite work of making sure your kid knows that you and your home are safe, affirming, and supportive. If you do ask, tell them that you heard it isn't helpful or wise to make assumptions about such things (you can even blame it on this book!). Make sure that you are able to say you love them regardless of their answer ("no matter what" is OK, but avoid saying, "even though").

**But the most important thing to do if you think your child might be LGB is showing them that you are the parent they can tell in their own time by showing that you love and accept them.**

Again, we can't make them who they are, but we can impact how they feel about who they are. If, as parents, you do some of these things, then—if your child is LGBT, they won't have to come out with fear and worry. It can just be about them being ready to share something important about themselves. And—if your kid is straight or cis, you will have taught them important lessons about openness, plurality, and equality. Win, win.

---

## LGBTW . . . Being Homophobic

I cannot stress this enough. If you are homophobic (or "homophobish") and you have a queer child in your life, please deal with it.

You can "disagree with" or "not believe in" homosexuality, queer relationships, or people being able to pee in bathrooms that do not necessarily match their genitalia all you want. You can be uncomfortable, you can be grossed out—whatever . . . your opinions are all your own.

The problem with homophobia is that those opinions tend to leak out beyond people's own, isolated thoughts and cause trouble in other people's lives—like prejudice, violence, loss of basic human rights or dignity and, sometimes, death.

The most common demographics in which homophobia is found are known.[1]

If you:

- are older,

- are male,

- don't have a college degree,

- are involved in organized religion,

- are supportive of traditional gender roles,

- lean politically conservative, and/or

- reside in an area where tolerance of same-sex marriage is low,

you are statistically more likely to be homophobic than the opposing counterparts (younger, educated, liberal, etc.).

Yes, I realize that you are already holding this book in your hands, and
I am therefore kicking at an open door, *and* this is still important. Because,
if you meet any of these criteria (and especially if you have someone in your
life who is important to you and who identifies as queer), please screen
yourself carefully and work on any un/conscious, internalized, or external-
ized homophobia.

These insidious (and typically irrational) fears and thoughts get in
the way of your relationships with the GLBT people in your life, and put
those people at risk for a whole slew of social damage, including lifelong
consequences (see chapter 34), and, sometimes, life-ending ones. In fact,
queer youth who come from rejecting families are eight times more likely
to attempt suicide than LGBT kids who have supportive families.[2]

Some of this can even be done by well-meaning family members in
ways that may not even be conscious, such as giving (or allowing other
family members to give) your child gifts, clothing, or activities that are
overtly stereotypical of their natal gender or sex, managing their gender-
atypicality by setting times and places where it is acceptable and times and
places where it is not, and assuming or acting as if their relationships with
friends of the opposite sex are romantic in nature (or forgetting that their
relationships with friends of the same natal sex could be).

One of the best "cures" for homophobia is having a person you already
know and love come out as queer. If you are homophobic/"homophobish,"
do not participate in the already caustic and inhospitable environment
many GLBT people face. Show them what it means to be human and that
you care.

There is much support and information to be found by and about other
parents and family members of queer youth.

**PFLAG.org** (Parents, Families and Friends of Lesbians and Gays)
supports equality and LGBTQ families, allies, and people through education and advocacy.

**FamilyProject.sfsu.edu**, The Family Acceptance Project, is a research, intervention, education, and policy initiative, based on the idea

that family acceptance of GLBT youth is a proven way to combat challenges like depression and suicide attempts, both of which disproportionately plague queer youth. They help ethnically, socially, and religiously diverse families support their LGBT children, through training, consultation, and crisis intervention.

## CHAPTER THIRTY-SEVEN
# IS MY CHILD TRANS?

I f you think your child may be trans or outside of the gender binary, there are some things to consider:

- Why do you think your child might be trans?

- Is this a gut feeling?

- Is this concern or idea coming from your child?

- Is this concern or idea coming from you?

- Is this concern or idea coming from others?

- Do strangers assume your son is a "girl" or your daughter a "boy"?

Trans kids can be remarkably open about their internal gender—especially when they are younger and not yet burdened with some of the cultural baggage we accumulate through age. It is common for people the child does not know to pick up on their true gender, "mistaking" them for the gender opposite to the one they were born. These more gut-level indicators can be more reliable signs of a child's gender identity than some of our own, sometimes-culturally-biased reactions to behaviors.

- Does your child gravitate toward games and topics not typical of their gender?

- Do they prefer to play with children of the opposite sex?

- Do they play *as* persons of the opposite sex or gender?

In addition to simply having gender atypical interests (as all children can), trans kids will also often gravitate toward peers of their true gender (a "boy" that chooses to play with cis girls or a "girl" who prefers to play with boys). Cis children tend to go through periods in which they will avoid playing (and even associating) with the opposite sex. Trans kids do not generally do this. Trans kids are also more likely to play at being the opposite gender in their pretend play. Does your son choose female video game avatars? Does your child insist on a gender-neutral nickname? Does your daughter prefer Superman, Luke Skywalker, or Harry Potter Halloween costumes over Wonder Woman, Princess Leia, or Hermione?

- Did you discover that your child has been cross-dressing?

- Is this something they do on occasion?

- Did they keep this secret or private?

- Was this a huge surprise to you?

Trans kids, especially at early ages, can be blissfully unaware of the "extraordinariness" of it all, and very matter-of-factly enter a men's bathroom, refuse to line up "with the girls" at preschool or simply explain, "I'm a girl, remember" or "you know I'm a boy, right?"—because, why wouldn't they? Cis children may experiment with clothing of the opposite sex (boys going through periods of wanting to wear princess dresses or girls refusing to wear dresses at all) or doing so as a joke or to be silly, but trans children prefer it.

- Have you discovered that your son has been stealing or borrowing women's clothes?

- Have they hid their desire to dress as the opposite sex from you?

- Was the focus only on lingerie?

Some straight and cis boys become fascinated with women's undergarments, whereas a trans kid would not typically focus only on undergarments—they are more likely interested in the entire presentation or outfit, not just the underthings.

Is your child uncomfortable, embarrassed, or do they rebel against their genitals (hiding or harming their penis or trying to pee standing up even though they do not have a penis)?

As I said above, there are variations in the ways that children express themselves, and of course none of this is necessarily concrete evidence one way or another—in fact if you live in a homo/transphobic household, family, religious community, or culture (in which accessing their true gender must be guised as a joke, kept private or hidden at all costs), then your answers to these questions may not provide any helpful information at all.

However, exploring these topics can provide some insight into your child, some clues to their gender identity and what next steps should be taken.

**If you think your child might be transgender:**

- Make sure your child knows that you respect their choices and take them seriously. Whether your child is gender dysphoric, trans, or their behavior truly is just a phase, parental support is crucial. No one ever died because they discussed gender with their children, bought them the clothes or toys they asked for, or let them steer their own ship regarding their gender presentation.

- Consult a professional well versed on the subject of gender.

**Gender dysphoria** is the medical diagnosis typically given to a person whose assigned birth gender is not the same as the one with which they identify.[1] Gender dysphoria used to be called gender identity disorder. As the problem is not a mental disorder, but the confusion, pain, and distress that the disconnect between a person's physical body and their internal sense of themselves can cause, it was changed. There is still some controversy about gender dysphoria being considered diagnosable like an illness, rather than a legitimate identity, though as a formal diagnosis it is still generally required in order to receive treatment and support for transitioning, and does enable access to medical care and resources.

Though it is true that some kids express gender nonconforming behavior throughout childhood and adolescence, and some may remain gender atypical or androgynous throughout their lifetime, some children do identify as a gender different than the one they were assigned at birth.

Being gender atypical is about how a child acts.

Being gender dysphoric is more about how a child *feels*.

So a gender dysphoric child both acts like *and* wants to *be* the opposite sex. More than just a boy wanting to wear dresses or not liking sports or a girl who likes to roughhouse with the neighbor boys instead of playing with dolls, gender dysphoric children express wanting to be the opposite sex or gender *in addition to* occasionally wanting to do some activities that our culture considers to be stereotypical of the other gender. In a sense—if you were to ignore the sex they were assigned at birth—they might show up quite gender (stereo) typical.

In contrast, the gender atypical kids—who express gender nonconforming behavior—will typically grow out of that behavior, and embrace the gender dress, demeanor, and deeds typical of their biology and the culture in which they are living sometime between five and ten years old. This is the developmental age at which they become conscious and clearer about the differences (both biological and cultural) between boys and girls, and find sticking their toes over those socially drawn lines uncomfortable.

The vast majority of children, even those who show up as gender atypical, will grow up to identify as straight and cis. Statistically, it appears right now that 3.5 percent of the populace will grow up to identify in the GLBT range,[2] with only 0.6 percent of the population growing up to identify as trans.[3]

Children develop in varying ways with a host of different temperaments, changes, and behaviors, and concepts of what is masculine or feminine also change. However, trans kids show up as much more obviously gender atypical *and* gender dysphoric than their non-trans counterparts. Trans girls can act in traditionally feminine ways: choosing to play with other girls, even walking or talking "like a girl." Trans boys, in contrast, may act in traditionally masculine ways, and are drawn to boys, boy games, and identify with boy heroes.

If a young child is both gender atypical *and* gender dysphoric, the chances of them eventually identifying as trans goes up. If a particular child reaches middle school age, and begins to realize that their body is starting to (or soon will) morph into something different than their internal concept, and they continue to display gender dysphoric statements and behaviors—then the chances of them growing to identify as trans also rises. In opposition to the gender atypical kids, above, what trans kids may find uncomfortable is *not* being able to stick their toes across those socially drawn lines—like not being able to use the "boys" restroom or to wear the "girls" graduation gown.

Here are some guidelines for discussing with your growing child whether they are transgender (rather than gender nonconforming or gender atypical)—ask if your child is:

- Consistent. Is your kid repeatedly gravitating toward a label or gender marker?

- Insistent. Is it the same label or gender marker or does it keep switching around?

- Persistent. Are they asking that others use that label or gender marker too?

If your child answered yes to these three questions, then it is important to find your child (and you) professional support and resources to explore next steps:

- GenderSpectrum.org's Parenting and Family page,

- transYouthEquality.org's For Parents page,

- PFLAG.org's Finding Support for You and Your Family page, and

- searching "Parenting transgender children" on social media sites like Facebook.

These resources can connect you with helpful people and information.

We are currently moving culturally much faster than the science or research around LGBT youth, and the choices we make (and don't make) about current generations will impact these processes for future ones.

Gender dysphoria and identity formation in children—both regarding their gender identity and their general sexuality—are really, really complicated things. How old does a child need to be before they know their true gender? When should trans kids be put on hormones? How young is too young? If my kid is gender atypical or gender dysphoric, what are the chances they will eventually identify as gay or trans? Assuming there is one blanket or correct answer to these questions is too simplistic, and makes it harder to ask and answer some of the other, more-important questions that need to be asked during these processes.

It is vital that gender atypical and dysphoric children be asked thoughtful, respectful questions about their experience, by parents who love them and professionals who understand sexuality, identity, and orientation. It is equally vital that their answers be listened to.

## CHAPTER THIRTY-EIGHT
# MY KID CAME OUT, NOW WHAT?

Understanding what LGBTQ is does not necessarily mean you understand your LGBTQ child. The reverse is also true: understanding your LGBTQ child does not necessarily mean you understand the dynamics involved in the life of an LGBTQ child.

We can be encouraged by the positive shifts in our cultural landscape, celebrating Pride events and anniversaries of positive milestones such as marriage equality in Massachusetts (2004). Pop culture and opinion polls have shown tangible evidence of GLBTQ equality.

This does not erase the facts that LGBTQ youth continue to suffer higher incidents of bullying, depression,[1] and are four times more likely to attempt suicide than their straight peers.[2] Kids who are not white or not cisgender have even higher rates,[3] and if their families reject them, that number doubles.[4]

Finding out your son or daughter is gay, lesbian, bisexual, or trans is not easy for anyone, and can be actively difficult for some.

Some parents are shocked when a child comes out; others see it coming. Some are welcoming; some are not. Some are supportive; others are not. One's reaction to the news when it is actually delivered can be unpredictable. Not all of our reactions are positive. Not all of our questions or even our well-intentioned bids are going to feel good to them.

And that's OK.

I coach kids that parents, friends, and other supportive important people in their lives get a year. A whole year to struggle, to wrap their brains around stuff, to slip up and say stupid things, to ask uncomfortable or even inappropriate questions.

One year.

Then it's time to get up, get over it, get on board.

In the meantime, you do what you have to do to keep them alive and in your home. Because supportive reactions help your kids cope (and helping them will eventually help you cope).

And here's a guide to help you.

## Ten Things *Not* To Do When Your Kid Comes Out to You

### Do not try to cure them.

Trying to change a person's gender identity—by any tactic, including denial, guilt, fear, force, or so-called reparative therapies, is not only ineffective, it is dangerous and can do permanent damage. In fact, those "conversion therapies," which are typically faith-based, have been wholly condemned as psychologically harmful by the American Psychological Association, the American Medical Association, the American Psychiatric Association, and numerous similar professional organizations.

### Do not say the word *phase*.

Phases are things, and young people *are* more prone to them than grown-ups, but phases revolve around things like certain bands, book series, or skinny jeans. Dismissing their gender identity as something fleeting like hair dye or how high to pull up your socks can be both insulting and harmful at a time when your child may need support the most.

### Do not make it about you.

Some parents feel guilt. Others feel fear. Some ask themselves, "Did I do (or *not* do) something to cause this?" Some worry about their child's health and welfare, wondering if it is somehow their "fault." Others' immediate response (and assumption) is that grandchildren are no longer an option. Thoughts like these are commonplace—but do not help. There is

---

### LGBTW . . . Grandchildren

Being LGBT does not mean your child can't be a parent, themselves, someday. Adoption, of course, is always an option, but natal males can bank sperm, and natal females can have their eggs frozen for later use, making biological children at least a future possibility.

---

a place for this angst and anxiety, and there are loads of resources, online and group supports as well as trained professionals to help you—don't put this on your kid. This is stuff you can talk about later, after you've worked through it and sorted it out.

### Do not refuse to acknowledge the issue.

Whether it's about gender or sexuality, things like refusing to use their name or pronouns or refusing to discuss significant others or invite them to family gatherings make them feel invisible. And invisible people get the message that they are supposed to disappear. . . .

### Do not assume that their experiences, desires, and choices will look like other gay, lesbian, bi, trans people you know or have heard about or seen on TV.

It's true that previous generations were sometimes forced or directed into narrow behaviors and lifestyles (like musical theater or priesthood), and now we have all these stereotypes to lug around (like the girls' gym coach with the clunky shoes and all those keys), but advancements in culture and technology have changed the rules, and anything is possible.

### Do not shield yourself from the visuals.

Some of the biggest issues in dealing with a queer child are the visual images! One of the reasons gay folks have had to work so hard to be accepted is because it is a *sexual* orientation, and just by its very nature, when it is mentioned or referenced, it conjures a visual. You may have given a passing thought to Brad and Angelina in the sack, casually considered Michelle and Barack "doing it" perhaps . . . but many of you, not until just now. Think about the last relative you had who got married. Did you visualize that particular couple actually having sex? Probably not. But for many people, when we hear about the lesbians who moved in down the street, or that cousin or nephew who just came out . . . we *see* it in a way that makes many people uncomfortable simply because it is more rare/different than our own experience.

## Do not forget about the extended family.

One of the biggest hurdles many queer kids (and their parents) have to deal with is the extended family. Many of us have parents who are still alive and kicking and saying awkward things in the grocery store or at Thanksgiving . . . sometimes we need to be the translator (or shield) between our children and that previous generation.

## Do not say "even though" when you tell them you love them. Do not be afraid to ask them questions and talk about it.

They are still the kid you have always known, and they want you to know them.

---

### LGBTW . . . Desensitization

It wasn't that long ago that things like showing Lucile Ball actually pregnant on television freaked viewers out. In the 1960 Uhura (black) and Captain Kirk (white) kissed on *Star Trek* and America freaked out. Carol and Mike Brady were the first couple on television to be shown in bed together. In the 1980s there was a plethora of shows (*Murphy Brown*, *Designing Women*, *Golden Girls*, *Kate & Allie*) in which women were shown living viable and independent lives as people, professionals, and parents without the necessity of men. In terms of the portrayal of queer characters in visual media, we have moved far and away from Klinger and Jack Tripper, the first two openly "queer" characters on prime time television—both of whom were pretending! Watching movies and television shows that show *actual* gay characters expressing affection and sexuality can help with your desensitization.

---

### Do not ask them questions and talk about it all of the time.

Their identity is a part of who they are, and though from time to time it may be the loudest or sparkliest . . . it is not the biggest part, nor the most important. . . .

## Ten Things to Do When Your Kid Comes Out to You

### Be proud of them.

Even just a generation ago, a queer child was much, much more likely to stifle, pretend, and stay closeted until they left home and went out on their own, before coming back home and coming out dramatically over Christmas dinner or the sixth night of Hanukkah. Be proud of yourself for raising a child with the insight and ego strength to identify something in them that some people aren't able to do until their twenties or thirties. Coming out at a young age shows a level of bravery and integrity that we should all aspire to.

### Understand your teen did not choose to be queer.

There may even be times when you may feel shocked or sad or even embarrassed or uncomfortable, and remembering that they may be feeling the exact same thing, through no fault of their own, can help you through those rough patches.

### Educate yourself and find support.

You are not alone. There are a number of organizations of parents of transgender children and teens, as well as individuals that support such parents.

### Accept them and always use your child's preferred gender pronouns and preferred names.

### Be your child's advocate.

Call out homo/transphobia when you see it, and demand that others respect your child's identity.

### Be there to help with any problems that arise.

Your pediatrician may be able to help you with this new challenge or suggest a referral for counseling. You also may find it helpful to talk with other parents whose children are lesbian, gay, or bisexual.

### Have your antennae (and speakers) tuned for violence.

Be watchful of behaviors that might indicate your child is a victim of bullying. If emotional or physical violence is suspected, ask them questions, and take immediate action—working with school personnel and other adults in the community.

### Ask for consent before outing them.

There is Pride and then there is the inappropriate sharing of personal information.

### Remember you have to come out, too.

Take your time, trust your gut. There is no timeline or recipe. There is no all or nothing. It is as incremental as it is important. *How* fast/often/thoroughly you come out to others about your queer kid is not as important as the fact that you are coming out.

### Mind the single sex situations.

Locker rooms, some team sports, or recreational activities and, yes, public restrooms are some (of the many) places or activities that require certain spacing or specific dress based on anatomy. Situations like these can be some of the most stressful and humiliating activities for queer kids—especially transgender kids. More inclusive or permeable activities, such as mixed sex choirs, art or technology classes (where nudity in locker rooms can be avoided), co-ed sports leagues, or things such as martial arts (where the uniforms are gender-neutral) can be much less stressful.

You may need to readjust your dreams for your child's future. You may have to deal with your own negative stereotypes of gay, lesbian, and bisexual people. You may need to protect them from grandma or the PTA's politics, you may even have to go back and clean up some jokes or comments you have made in the past.

See above re: That's OK / One year. But, get on with it.

Because parental support predicts greater mental and physical health, including higher self esteem, and lower substance abuse. Because, your support protects against depression and homelessness—at which GLBTQ youth are already higher risk. And because, for many LGBT youth, the support of their family can, literally, be the difference between life and death.

## CHAPTER THIRTY-NINE
# THE FAMILY THAT TRANSITIONS TOGETHER . . .

Transgender youth particularly are invisible in many ways in today's modern culture, because in most of Western society a binary (two-part) classification of gender is assumed to be the norm. In a binary-biased culture, people are expected to assume the gender identity of their biological sex, including all of the expectations and roles associated with that sex/gender. Most people are classified as male or female, and people who show or have characteristics typically reserved for the other gender are viewed as different and treated badly.

Developing and integrating a positive gender identity is a developmental task for all adolescents. For trans youth, however, there is the additional challenge of integrating their (sometimes complex) gender identity with their biological body, but also their larger, family, ethnic, and cultural backgrounds.

Not only is adolescence a time of change in both physical appearance and self-concept, but we live in a society that places a massive amount of importance on appearance.

If you take the time, it is not difficult to understand what it means to be living in a body that is incongruent to how you know and understand yourself.

For a trans kid, pubertal changes, that cis children may be excited about, are experienced as more stressful than their non-trans peers. Parents who are cisgender and/or may not accurately remember the throes of their own puberty may not understand how deeply disturbing this process can be.

To wrap your brain around this concept, try to understand that for a trans girl, her voice deepening or growing facial hair would be just as traumatic as it would be for a natal girl. Similarly, a trans boy who started to develop breasts or have a period might feel as humiliated as a natal boy would.

Many gender dysphoric children feel extremely uncomfortable wearing clothing that is especially iconic of their birth sex; for example, a trans boy may feel mortified if required to wear feminine dresses or makeup, in exactly the same manner as a natal boy who was forced to wear such clothing.

Clothing specifically designed for anatomical reasons can also be traumatizing and shaming for trans kids to wear, such as a trans girl being made to wear a boy's bathing suit, or a trans boy being expected to wear a two-piece bathing suit.

Everyone has the right to feel and look the way they want to look, to figure out and appreciate who they are meant to be, to navigate puberty and adolescence with as little drama and trauma as possible, and to be able to represent their identity and gender accurately to the world.

## Social Transition

Every child, family, and situation is unique. There is no right or wrong way to help your child socially transition. It is important to be patient with anyone who is questioning or exploring their gender identity. Our gender identity is one of the basic building blocks of our core selves, and it is natural that someone who is questioning or exploring their gender identity may take some time to sort out how best to explore their identity and express their gender.

Trial runs (in which you allow your child to live as their true gender, with a different name and their desired pronouns for a predetermined period of time such as a weekend or a brief vacation) can be an excellent way to help your child begin their social transition, in a fun and less-stressful way. They can interact with people who do not know they are trans, and experimenting with temporary transitions will give your child a taste of the freedom and identity they want, plus, social transition can also be a way for your child to clarify that this is, indeed, what they want.

### Home

You and other family members may feel awkward using a new name and gender for your trans kid. This takes time. They might even choose a new name or pronoun, and then decide later to change one or both of them. The most important thing is to practice, do your best to use the name and/or pronoun requested, and set an expectation in the house of apologies (and graciousness) when someone misses the mark.

## School

Do not let your child's school sabotage their social transition.

Many schools may be inexperienced or unprepared to support a trans child. In these situations the bulk of their education about the subject may fall, unfortunately, upon your shoulders.

Some schools may single your child out by trying to dictate what bathrooms your child uses, where they change for swim practice, which team they are practicing for, where they sleep on class or team trips, or what color gown they wear at graduation.

Even well-intentioned schools may make a trans student's school life stressful. Some schools may ironically try to make a trans student feel more comfortable by "celebrating" them, over (or overtly) acknowledging them as part of the community, outing them, and/or drawing uncomfortable attention to their "differentness."

It is vital that your child be treated and regarded as actually being a member of his/her new and chosen gender/sex.

If you do not believe that your child can or should socially transition in their school or your house, because of social or safety issues, consider other options such as family or friends who might be able to take your child in for a period of time or changing schools once their social transition is underway.

## Finding a Therapist

Trans kids do not need professional counseling, therapy, or other intervention simply because they are trans. There is nothing inherently disordered about being gender atypical. Transitioning is a healthy and rational response to that dynamic. But a well-versed and competent professional can make your child's (and your family's) transition smoother.

If you do seek professional help, it is critical that you make sure you find a therapist, psychologist, clinic, or clinician specializing in gender dysphoria in children. Some professionals believe that transgender children are disordered and should/can be "fixed." This is extremely dangerous.

Connecting your child to age-appropriate resources in your community during their social transition will help them find and maintain friendships with other trans kids of similar age, help them evolve into their identity, and give them the sense that they fit in.

## Medical Transition

Some families opt for hormone replacement therapy (HRT) (see chapter 12) during the teen years; others choose to wait until later teens or adulthood. Puberty blockers are another option. There are benefits and drawbacks with each, and your doctor or a therapist can help you sort out which path is best for your child and family.

As soon as you become aware that your child is trans, you should begin preparing financially for the possibility of future, medical expenses.

Review your healthcare insurance options. HRT, gender confirmation surgery, or other procedures associated with medical transition can be quite expensive, and financially difficult without the help of insurance.

Even for those with insurance, not all policies cover these procedures, or do not have structures in place to cover gender specific issues for transgender people—such as someone with a male gender marker (but who has an intact, female reproductive system) not being able to have things like birth control, or gynecological care covered because they are a man.

More and more companies are beginning to acknowledge that there is a diversity in bodies and identity, though many still require people to check either the "male" or "female" box, ignore the larger context, and some even have language written into their policies that is specifically exclusive of transgender people and issues.

At some point your child may ask for or require surgeries or other medical procedures. In the hospital, insisting that your child have either a room to themselves, or with another trans kid of the same social gender and sexual orientation will likely make your child more comfortable.

### After Transition

It is natural (especially after having your child in the hospital) to feel protective. Some parents are tempted to limit their child's social circle and activities to only those friends who are aware of their trans status. Other parents are tempted to inform or educate their child's friend's parents—in effect "outing" them before they may be ready. It is important, during this time, to discuss with your child what kind of support they want and need, and how they would like you to support them.

Keep an eye out for signs of depression, which can be a normative reaction after the anticipation and excitement and exhaustion associated with surgical procedures.

Parenting any teenager is both challenging and rewarding. Taking time for self-care is always important, but seeking support for yourself as a parent of an LGBT kid can be even more necessary. Friends, therapists, support groups, online resources (such as forums, blogs, or social media), and books like this one, can clear up confusion and combat the isolation that some parents of LGBT kids face.

# PARENTING YOUR QUEER KID

Almost in opposition to hateful or unsupportive parents who cut off or disown their child, sometimes loving and well-intentioned parents are reluctant to criticize, say no, or set limits for fear of coming across as intolerant, alienating, or accidentally oppressing their children.

There *are* some unique dynamics in parenting an GLBT child, but queer kids crave structure and need boundaries just as much as any other kid.

In many ways, it's important (even wise) to treat your kid as you would any other kid their age, and communication is key—not just about sexuality, gender, safety, and politics, but boundaries, rules and respect, curfews, and chores. . . .

## Queer-Specific Questions Parents Often Have

### How do I talk about this stuff if I'm not LGBT?

Being familiar with gay sexuality, relationships, and—yes, even the sex—before engaging your teen in discussions about sexuality will help you be prepared for questions and advice.

Talking about sex with a straight kid can be a little more obvious and straight-forward (no pun), but with gay kids, there are a range of things out there that they will need to prepare for that are outside your experience and that don't even relate to the things they hear about sex from their straight friends or classes at school.

### How do I talk about the sex, specifically?

Generally, the safer sex rules and guidelines apply. There are not a lot of specific resources out there, but Scarleteen.org and the book you are holding are two of the best. They can give you some guidelines on how to talk about safer sex concepts including abstinence. It's true, most of the initialism (LGB) *is* about sexual orientation, but that does not mean that LGB youth are any less likely or able to choose to wait to become sexually active. There may be an assumption (either on their part or yours) that since they are out about their sexual orientation that sexual behavior must necessarily be the next step. Even if you and your child consult reliable resources, discussions about safer sex, STIs, consent, intimate partner violence, sexual assault, and even pregnancy still need to happen.

Thoughts of our adolescent children as sexual beings may make us uncomfortable, but visions of them tumbling down flights of stairs as toddlers spurred us to have safety conversations back then. The thought of them putting themselves through car windshields motivates us to teach them how to navigate intersections and freeways when behind the wheel. If discussion about how to navigate their genitals is different, it is quite likely because of our own discomfort with the subject matter, and that's a poor reason to avoid the topic.

---

## LGBTW . . . Tips for Talking About Sex and Sexuality

- Make the subject a regular topic of conversation. It is not a one-time inoculation, it is a process. Information on how to use this book as a resource can be found in the Outro that follows this chapter.

- Find teachable moments and include sex whenever you talk about dating, love, drugs, friendship, health, media, and other related subjects. Do it every chance you get. Bringing it up at the dinner table may not be a good idea, but song lyrics, websites, movies, newscasts, and the like can be excellent opportunities for the topics to come up.

- Keep the lines of communication open. You'll need to discuss tough topics from time to time. If you and your teen are used to having conversations on a regular basis, even the awkward conversations will be easier. You don't want to think about

---

them as sexually active creatures any more than they want to picture you as one. Sleep safe in the knowledge that even if your kids might be uncomfortable talking to you, they know they can.

- Respect your child's opinions. Enjoy the fact that your children are curious and have begun to think for themselves. Work to form a relationship with those opinions—even when they don't mesh with your own.

- If you cannot have the discussion with them, provide them with reliable and responsible alternatives, such as caring adults who can.

- Speak to your child's school about what it is teaching and the sexual education curriculum, and do not assume that what your children are learning about sex outside your home is enough.

## How do I handle their boyfriend/girlfriend?

The same way you'd treat an opposite-sex boyfriend or girlfriend. Make an effort to get to know them. Discuss their goals and interests. Invite them to dinner. Get to know their parents if possible, or at least make contact.

On that same note, hold them to the same standards you would a cis/straight suitor. Do they want to meet you? Actively avoid you? Make sure they treat your teen with respect and kindness.

## What if their boyfriend/girlfriend is not out?

If your child's boyfriend or girlfriend has not come out to their parents, it's important to explore why. Their fears could be unfounded and unnecessary or about a fear of violence or of being kicked out of their house. It's not your job to out them or encourage them to, but advice and support are very human responses.

## But, does my kid seem *too* queer?

For some people, when they come out and become comfortable with themselves for the first time, they may have a tendency to behave in ways

---

### LGBTW . . . PDA

It's important to accept that teens experiment with their identity in all sorts of ways, and that queer kids, like straight/cis kids, will get crushes, get their hearts broken, date, and learn how to function in relationships, and about themselves in the process. And you will be witness to all of it. That being said, even if you like their boyfriend/girlfriend, seeing them holding hands or kissing may make you uncomfortable.

"Would this bother me in an opposite-sex partner?" is an important question to ask. If not, you may need to look past it, and try to connect with your teen's partner the best you can.

Another question is, "Is there something about the behavior that is *not* about the gender or sexuality that is troubling me?" If so, having a clarifying conversation with your kid is the next best step.

---

you might think are over the top. Perhaps it is about making up for lost time, about trying on a new aspect of their personality, about pride, politics, or just a normative developmental stage in their process, but there can be a period of time when your child's dress, demeanor, and deeds are loudly, obviously, and even stereotypically queer. Shocking or dramatic hairstyles, anger-fueled political arguments, and big, giant rainbow beach towels are not unusual during this process. Your kid's LGBTQness is not the largest or most important thing about them, but for a period of time, for their own emotional and social development, it may the loudest or sparkliest, and that's OK.

---

### LGBTW . . . "The 'Phobe Card"

They are teenagers—they will still want to go places or with people you do not approve. They will still wear clothing inappropriate to the weather or occasion. They will still want to watch or do things that are age inappropriate.

There may be times, with a queer kid, when there is a debate of some kind, a consequence or a difference of opinion and in the heat of battle the, "You're just being a homo/transphobe!" bomb is dropped on you.

It is very important when this happens:

---

- To make sure we are doing due diligence in terms of self-examination and are making sure that our own homo/trans-phobia is *not* the issue (because sometimes it is).

- To make sure we are separating who they are from what they do—that we are commenting on a behavior/pattern—not making a global statement about who they are as a person.

- To screen our statements and make sure that our stance would be / is the same for a straight/cis kid.

If you pass that litmus test,

- Do not back down or abdicate.

- Call B.S.

- Up the communication and clearly explain to them that it is not about their gender or orientation, but about their choices—because teaching our children to make good choices as teens is integral to learning to make good choices as an adult.

## How do I handle their friends?

Your child's relationships with their friends may take on a different tone once your kid is out as queer. If you wouldn't let a fifteen-year-old girl spend the night in your fifteen-year-old straight/cis son's room, or a fifteen-year-old boy spend the night in your fifteen-year-old straight/cis daughter's room, then you may find yourself uncomfortable with a fifteen-year-old gay/lesbian child who wants a same sex friend to stay over. If your trans daughter's inner friend circle is comprised of natal girls, do overnights with them make sense? What about your gay son and his straight best girlfriend? Your lesbian daughter and her gay BFF?

You may not feel comfortable with overnights with potential romantic partners, or them hanging out in their room with the door closed. You may insist on only group sleepovers or only slumber parties in the living room. You may also be fine with them spending the night, or having unsupervised time with potential partners. Whatever your stance, it is still

---

## LGBTW . . . Other People's Queer Kids

As hard as it may be to imagine—especially if you are doing your own work to be a supportive and loving parent of a queer kid—some parents of LGBT kids do not love and support their child, finding their queerness, identity, or orientation to be too much to handle.

Research shows that 40 percent of queer youth are disowned by, or run away from, their disapproving families as teenagers and end up as homeless.[1] These kids are very difficult to place in foster or group care, when programs are too often ill-equipped or unprepared to responsibly serve queer youth—who are disproportionately impacted by things such as homelessness, school push-out, substance abuse, and violence and do not have access to the same supports and services that other minorities have.

If you have room in your heart and your home, please consider fostering a queer kid, through your local child protective service agency. Caring and well-intentioned foster parents are always in demand—but especially those who are able (and willing) to support GLBT youth.

---

important to hold it purposefully, discuss house rules, and (again) not do anything you wouldn't do with a straight/cis kid.

### What if I don't trust my kid?

If you don't trust your teen, it's important to examine why. It may be completely justified, based on their past behavior, having nothing to do with their gender or sexuality. Or it might. Many GLBT youth have learned to develop muscles for flying under the radar or living less-than honestly as a natural defense mechanism or survival skill. If this is true for your child, and it continues once they are out, it is something that needs to be discussed and actively worked on. This will benefit both your relationship with them and their relationship with the world.

## Advocating for Your Child

As you step forward to help your child navigate the difficult job of growing up LGB or T, you will be judged by others: family and church members, insensitive friends and neighbors, ignorant school staff, hateful strangers, and the larger media culture.

You will feel the fear, anger, and bile from people, just like your child will. Your child did not choose this. But you will, because that is what parents do. We stand up, we stand in-between our child and the oncoming threat, we advocate, and we do not put up with others treating our child as less-than.

Of course, we cannot wrap our children in diapers and bubble wrap—they need to learn how to deal with such adversity themselves, but we can intervene at times to offer support and modeling and the sense that they never have to do this alone.

**Here are some tips:**

### Develop a relationship with your child's school.

There should be zero-tolerance for bullying. There should be a Gay/Queer Straight Alliance available as a resource. There should be no excuse-making for the mistreatment of LGBT students. In the absence of obviously supportive faculty and policy (or the presence of unsupportive faculty or policy), your influence with school administrators may be crucial.

### Do not let your child drop out of school to avoid bullying.

Too many queer youth drop out and never return. Transferring to a new school may be necessary or helpful in some situations (such as social transition), though it is important that a move such as that is a move toward something, rather than moving from something. It is important to make sure that the message your child takes away is not that *they* need to change. The school/bully needs to change. If they can or will not, then the circumstance does.

### Remember to keep an eye on your queer child's sibling/s.

Siblings of queer kids may need some extra support during transition.

- Having a sibling come out may bring up questions about their own gender identity or sexual orientation.

- They may mourn the loss of their sibling (of one orientation/gender) or need help navigating a different relationship with their sibling (of a new orientation/ gender).

- They may be negatively affected by relocations, school transfers, or room reassignments within the home.

- They may be worried and scared for their siblings as they go through coming out, and social and medical transition (having a sibling in the hospital can be particularly stressful).

- They may need support with feelings of confusion, fear, jealousy, or even resentment.

- They may now *also* be or feel "out" in places such as school, and can feel self-conscious, protective of their sibling, or have to navigate rumors and phobes in their own social circles. They too can be actively bullied or targeted because of their relationship to their GLBT sibling. Some of those siblings may also turn to bullying or bashing as a way of winning social approval or avoiding negative, social targeting, which can permanently damage the sibling relationship.

Listening, a bit of extra love and attention, as well as professional counseling can be especially helpful in these situations.

### Communication is key with regard to co-parenting.

Each family's growth, dynamics, and process can be different. Of course, supporting your child should ideally be your top priority as a parent, but it is understandable that there may be a disconnect between intention and execution. Life happens, other things may need to take precedence on occasion, and different parents having different types of reactions is not uncommon—especially when parents are not (or never were) married to each other. Bringing an experienced professional into the conversation can help incorporate everyone's needs into the equation, facilitate less-awkward and uncomfortable conversation, and provide a framework for teamwork.

### Become a professional Ally.

Seek out queer culture in your community. Check out books, films, YouTube channels, and blogs to find out more about LGBT lives. Model using your own pronouns when you introduce yourself to people. Throw some bumper stickers on your car. Be visible on social media. Vote with your child's best interests in mind.

Do whatever you can, however small, to help the queer youth in your life feel safe, supportive, and successful.

# OUTRO

## For Parents

Sexual education that serves and includes GLBT youth involves particular and unique dynamics and information. The assumptions and eliminations inherent in typical, mainstream, abstinence-only education prevent GLBT students from learning the information and skills they need to stay healthy, and contribute to a climate of exclusion in schools (where LGBT students are already frequent targets of bullying and discrimination).

This means helping our kids create boundaries, grow, and reinforce their decision-making skills, and starting conversations about values with regard to sex and sexuality are likely going to fall on your shoulders.

As a parent myself, and as someone who has worked with teens for almost twenty years, I believe that knowledge and self-confidence are the best protection against the unfortunate consequences that sometimes accompany sexual activity. Teaching children about healthy sexuality while they are still open to adult influence spares us from witnessing them putting themselves at risk later in life because of a lack of knowledge.

I wrote this book with the intention of providing information, education, and inspiration in order to contribute to healthy social and sexual relationships. This book can be left in an accessible place, such as a bookshelf, desktop, coffee table, or waiting room of a health professional—somewhere low-key where a teen can discover it and read it in private. Parents can write notes in the margins and quietly leave it on an underager's nightstand, inviting them to ask questions, or they can read it chapter by chapter with their daughters, planning discussions afterward. Therapists and teachers can use it as an educational guideline for groups.

## For Readers

For the young people reading this, this book is designed to give you the tools and knowledge that you need to develop a relationship with your self, sex and sexuality, and expression—being healthy and having fun while doing as little harm to yourself and others as possible.

I strongly encourage anyone reading this to seek adult support and professional help if

- you are just becoming sexually active,

- your sexual behavior is causing problems in your life,

- your sexual behavior is causing problems in others' lives,

- you might be (or have gotten someone) pregnant,

- you fear you have been exposed to infection,

- you have a history of abuse,

- you are afraid of your sexual or romantic partner,

- you have a history of self-harming behaviors,

- you have questions about your sexual or gender identity,

- you experience barriers to expressing your sexual or gender identity,

- you feel unsafe, unsupported, or actively bullied because of your sexual identity.

This book is intended to provide information, education, and inspiration. It is intended to be an adjunct to, not a substitute for, professional medical or legal advice. Laws and practices vary state-by-state, region-by-region, country-by-country. In addition, much of the information included here can and (most likely) will change with time and with the rapid development of technology, science, and culture. It is in your best interest to confirm any content inside (and its relevance to your own life and circumstance) by doing your own research.

I value feedback and questions, and I strive to respond. I can be reached via my website, beheroes.net.

# GLOSSARY

**ABORTION** Ending the life of a developing fetus via a number of techniques.

**ABSTINENCE** Choosing to not participate in sex and sexual play with other people.

**ACE** Shortened version of **ASEXUAL**.

**ACQUIRED IMMUNE DEFICIENCY SYNDROME** When a person's immune system is considered too compromised (too weak) to keep them safe from bacterial and viral infections that they would normally be able to fend off.

**ACTIVISM** Working with other people and groups in one's community to motivate political and social justice and change.

**ADOLESCENCE** The transition between childhood and adulthood.

**AFTERPLAY** All of the fun, lovey, gropey stuff you do after the *actual* sex.

**THE AGE RULE** A formula to ensure that one engages in sexual/romantic relationships with people within their general cohort.

**AGENDER** Identifying as neither male nor female and/or rejecting the idea of a gender binary altogether.

**AIDS** (see **ACQUIRED IMMUNE DEFICIENCY SYNDROME**).

**ALTERNATIVES** A natural, contraceptive / safer sex method involving the penetration of orifices other than the vagina—such as the mouth or anus.

**ANAL SEX** (PENIS-ANUS) When a person inserts their penis into the anus of another person.

**ANALINGUS** Putting one's mouth on someone's anus.

**ANDROGYNY** Having both traditionally masculine and feminine qualities, or qualities that do not fit cleanly into typical masculine and feminine roles.

**ANUS** The opening of the rectum, which is also highly sensitive to touch and can provide sexual pleasure.

**ASEXUALITY** A sexual orientation characterized by a lack of sexual interest, desire, or activity.

**AUGMENTATION MAMMOPLASTY** A top surgery for MTF trans people involving the enlargement of breast tissue.

**BALLS** (see **TESTICLES**).

**BEING TRANSPARENT** (see **PASSING**).

**BI** Shortened version of **BISEXUAL**.

**BI PRIVILEGE** The benefit and advantages a bi person may experience because their sexual orientation is not known, discovered, or obvious.

**BINDING** A method of social transition involving flattening one's breasts in order to create a more male-like chest and curb dysphoria in FTM trans people.

**BIOLOGY** The physical makeup of the human body—its parts and functions.

**BISEXUALITY** Some degree of attraction to both sexes.

**BLENDING** (see **PASSING**).

**BLOW JOB** (see **FELLATIO**).

**BODY IMAGE** The way we see ourselves in our minds and mirrors, and the ways we feel about that.

**BONER** (see **ERECTION**).

**BONER SHAME** Anxiety around the size of one's penis.

**BOTTOM** The person being penetrated during anal sex.

**BOTTOM SURGERY** A method of medical transition that involves either feminizing or masculinizing a trans person's internal and external genitalia.

**BREAST SELF-EXAM** Checking for lumps, bumps, or changes in the breasts as a preventative screen for cancer.

**BREASTS** Mammary glands, which secrete milk used to feed infants, are sensitive to touch and can enhance sexual pleasure.

**BUTT PLUG** A dildo specifically designed for insertion into an anus.

**CASTRATION** A bottom surgery for MTF trans people involving the removal of the testicles and most of the penis.

**CASUAL SEX** Sexual activity without romantic connection.

**CERVICAL CAP** A custom-fitted, thimble-shaped, latex cap, which covers the cervix and prevents the passage of sperm.

**CERVICAL SHIELD** A silicone cup attached to the cervix via suction, which covers the cervix, and prevents the passage of sperm.

**CERVIX** A small, doughnut-shaped organ, which connects the uterus and the back of the vagina.

**CHANCROID** Sexually transmitted bacterium in the form of small, pus-filled, and painful ulcers on the genitals.

**CHEST RECONSTRUCTION** A top surgery for FTM trans people involving the removal of breast tissue.

**CHLAMYDIA** A bacterium which causes painful and burning discharges during urination and intercourse, inflammation of the rectum and cervix, swelling of the testicles, bleeding after sex and, eventually, sterility.

**CIRCUMCISION** A controversial surgical procedure in which the foreskin is cut off or removed from a penis.

**CISGENDER** An umbrella term used to describe people whose gender identity (sense of themselves as male or female) or gender expression is in line with the parts they were born with (or acquire later through surgery).

**CLITORIS** A short shaft with a very sensitive tip, the only female organ whose sole purpose is pleasure—it plays an incredibly important part in sexual arousal.

**CLOCKED** The opposite of passing, meaning having been recognized as a transgender person.

**CLOSETED** The opposite of being out as a gay person.

**COCK** (see **PENIS**).

**COERCION** When someone does something someone does not like in order to get them to go along with unwanted sexual contact.

**COME** (see **SEMEN**).

**COMING** (see **EJACULATION**).

**COMING OUT** The process of accepting and being open about one's sexual orientation and gender identity.

**CONDOM RESISTANCE TECHNIQUES** Tactics used to convince a partner to not use a condom.

**CONDOMS (FEMALE)** Longer, wider form of male condoms, inserted into the vagina or rectum and held in place with bendable rings at both ends.

**CONDOMS (MALE)** Latex coverings placed on the penis to prevent sperm from entering the vagina, anus, or mouth.

**CONSENT** On-purpose, sober, chosen, informed, mutual, honest, and obvious agreement.

**CONTRACEPTIVES** Technology and medications (such as pills, patches, and devices) that reduce the likelihood of pregnancy.

**CONVERSION THERAPY** Ineffective and harmful use of prayer, counseling, and sometimes drugs or shock therapy meant to "cure" gay people.

**CRABS** Tiny, gray bugs that attach to your skin, turn darker when swollen with blood, and attach eggs to your pubic hair.

**CROSS-DRESSER** (see **TRANSVESTITE**).

**CUM** (see **SEMEN**).

**CUMMING** (see **EJACULATION**).

**CUNNILINGUS** Oral sex on a vagina.

**DATE RAPE DRUGS** Chemicals usually put into someone's drink, which weaken you and impair your ability to move or remember things.

**DATING VIOLENCE** Abusive, aggressive, and controlling behavior in a relationship.

**DEATH GRIP** Masturbating too quickly and/or with a very tight grip.

**DENTAL DAMS** Ultra-thin, often scented, latex sheets placed over the vulva or anus during oral sex.

**DEPO-PROVERA** A once-per-three-months birth control injection.

**DESIRE** Interest in sex and sexual behavior / feeling attracted to someone.

**DETUMESCE** The opposite of erection.

**DIAPHRAGM** A shallow rubber cup, which covers the cervix to prevent the passage of sperm.

**DICK** (see **PENIS**).

**DIGITAL ABUSE** Using tech or the Internet to harass someone else. Things like invading privacy, bullying, threatening, unwanted images or messages and cyberstalking would fall into this category.

**DIGITAL CITIZENSHIP** The cultural rules and customs of appropriate, mannerly, responsible and safe behavior online and through screens.

**DILDO** Wood, glass, metal, plastic or rubber masturbatory devices, similar to vibrators, though lacking the vibration aspects, and often shaped to look like an actual penis.

**DOUCHE** (A) A mix of water, fragrances, and chemical cleaning agents inserted into a vagina for irrigation. (B) A sanitary choice some people make before anal sex in which they irrigate their rectum with water. (C) Those guys (they tend to be male-identified) who obviously and purposely think themselves too hip, too sexy, and (try) too much, stinking up the room with faux and forced charm, pseudo-macho selfishness, and self-promotion.

**DRAG KING** Females who live part-time as members of the other sex, primarily as performers—singing and/or dancing.

**DRAG QUEEN** Males who live part-time as members of the other sex, primarily as performers—singing and/or dancing.

**DRY SEX** (see **OUTERCOURSE**).

**DYKE** Offensive term for lesbians.

**ECPs** (see **EMERGENCY CONTRACEPTION PILLS**).

**EGGS** Contain the female DNA and twenty-three chromosomes, which (if joined by the male DNA and twenty-three chromosomes of a sperm) create an embryo.

**EJACULATION** The discharge of fluids from vaginas and penises, usually during orgasm.

**EMBRYO** A human organism in the early stages of development.

**EMERGENCY CONTRACEPTION PILLS** Increased doses of birth control hormones used by some as a backup when other means of contraception have failed.

**EMOTIONAL ABUSE** Threats, insults, intimidation and isolation, or stalking.

**ERECTION** A penis engorged with blood and "hard."

**EROGENOUS ZONES** Areas which, when stimulated, can lead to high levels of sexual arousal and powerful orgasms.

**ESSURE** Small, (non-surgical) metallic implants inserted into the fallopian tubes to block pregnancy.

**EXCITEMENT** Feeling actively turned on or engaged in sexual activity.

**FACEBOOK DEPRESSION** When comparing oneself to others' cool blogs or profiles, others' friends and followers, others' posts, pictures, bodies, lives and likes, leaves one feeling more and more crappy about oneself.

**FAG/FA.FERTILITY AWARENESS METHODS** (see **RHYTHM METHODS**).

**FERTILIZATION** The fusion of the sperm and egg.

**FETUS** A human organism after eight weeks of development, when recognizable human characteristics begin to show.

**FLACCID** A penis when it is not erect or "hard."

**FOMO** An acronym for the Fear Of Missing Out; that creepy feeling we sometimes get when we are not plugged into our devices and we sense that something-cool-or-important-is-happening-somewhere-and-I-am-missing-it!

**FOREPLAY** All the fun, lovey, gropey stuff you do before the *actual* sex.

**FORESKIN** A retractable, double-layered, fold of skin that covers and protects the glans of the penis when it is not erect.

**FRENCH KISSING** Opening the mouth and putting your tongue in the other person's mouth (or letting them do that to yours).

**FRENULUM** The sensitive area under the head of the penis.

**FRIENDS-WITH-BENEFITS (FWB)** Sexual, but not romantic, relationships between otherwise platonic friends.

**GARDASIL** A vaccine that prevents the types of the Human Papillomavirus (HPV), which can cause cervical cancer and genital warts.

**GAY** A male who is attracted to another male.

**GAYCISM** (see **HOMODIUM**).

**GENDER** A social phenomenon, often used to refer to ways that people act, interact, or feel about themselves, which are associated with boys'/men and girls/women. This refers to how "guy-like" or "chick-like" one is.

**GENDER DYSPHORIA** Feelings of confusion, pain, and anxiety caused by the disconnect between a person's physical body and their internal sense of themselves.

A medical diagnosis referring to the distress felt by a person whose assigned birth gender is not the same as the one with which they identify.

**GENDER EXPRESSION** One's dress, demeanor, and deeds, the relationship of those things to one's sexual and gender identity, and how those things are interpreted by others.

**GENDER IDENTITY** One's sense of oneself as male, female, both, or neither. Trans(gender) or Cis(gender) can be descriptors of this phenomenon.

**GENDER IDENTITY DISORDER** Outdated diagnostic term (see **GENDER DYSPHORIA**).

**GENDERQUEER** Being a third sex—both male *and* female—and/or falling completely outside the gender binary (e.g., genderless—being neither male nor female).

**GENITALS** Reproductive body parts.

**GENITAL WARTS** (see **HPV**).

**GLANS** The sensitive "head" of the penis.

**GONORRHEA** A bacterium that causes sterility, arthritis, heart problems, and a pus-like discharge from the urethra, which causes pain during urination.

**GRÄFENBERG SPOT** A female erogenous zone located inside the vagina.

**GROOMING** When someone does something someone likes in order to get them to go along with unwanted sexual contact.

**GROWER** A shorter, soft penis that increases, sometime doubling or tripling in length, as it gets erect.

**GSA** (Gay Straight Alliance) Extracurricular, school-sponsored support and recreational clubs for queer youth and their allies (see **QSA**).

**G-SPOT** (see **GRÄFENBERG SPOT**).

**GYNE** (see **VAGINA**).

**GYNECOLOGY** The study and treatment of the female reproductive system.

**HARD-ON** (see **ERECTION**).

**HEPATITIS B** A very contagious virus that attacks the liver, leading to yellow skin, brown urine cirrhosis, cancer, and possibly death.

**HERMAPHRODITE** A stigmatizing word for intersexed persons, which should not be used to refer to people.

**HERPES SIMPLEX 1** Cold sores or fever blisters around the mouth.

**HERPES SIMPLEX 2** Hot, itchy blisters, which burst open and create ulcers around the genital areas.

**HETEROSEXUAL** Romantic or sexual attraction to someone of the opposite sex.

**HICKEYS** Bruises caused by sucking blood to the surface of the skin.

**HIV** (see **HUMAN IMMUNODEFICIENCY VIRUS**).

**HOMODIUM** Targeted hatred and chosen disgust toward gay people and culture.

**HOMOPHOBIA** Discrimination and fear against gay people and culture.

**HOMOSEXUAL** Romantic or sexual attraction to someone of the same sex.

**HOOKUP** Sexual interactions that happen spontaneously between people who just met or do not know each other well (see **ONE-NIGHT STAND**).

**HORMONE REPLACEMENT THERAPY** A method of medical transition involving the prescription and use of hormones that develop secondary sex characteristics.

**HORNY** (see **DESIRE**).

**HPV** (see **HUMAN PAPILLOMAVIRUS**).

**HRT** (see **HORMONE REPLACEMENT THERAPY**).

**HUMAN IMMUNODEFICIENCY VIRUS** A viral STI, which slowly weakens your immune system—your body's mechanism for fighting off infections.

**HUMAN PAPILLOMAVIRUS** Cell-mutating viruses that cause a variety of itchy, flesh-colored, cauliflower-like warts, some of which also contribute to cancers in the cervix, vulva, and penis.

**HUMAN TRAFFICKING** When someone is forced to do sexual things in order to make money, such as forced prostitution, being kidnapped into "sex slavery," or making someone pose for pornographic pictures.

**HVB** (see **HEPATITIS VIRUS B**).

**HYMEN** A thin piece of tissue that partially covers the opening of the vagina.

**HYSTERECTOMY** A bottom surgery for FTM trans people in which the uterus and ovaries are removed.

**IDENTITY** The who or what someone is or wishes to be known as.

**INDULGENCE** The decision whether or not to remain abstinent.

**INTERSEX** A person having biological characteristics of both the male and female sexes or who is chromosomally (internally) one sex, while physically (externally) another.

**INTRAUTERINE DEVICE** A small, plastic, T-shaped device inserted into the woman's uterus containing copper, which helps prevent the fertilization and implantation of eggs.

**INTRAUTERINE SYSTEM** A small, plastic, T-shaped device inserted into the woman's uterus containing hormones, which help prevent the fertilization and implantation of eggs.

**IUD** (see **INTRAUTERINE DEVICE**).

**IUS** (see **INTRAUTERINE SYSTEM**).

**JACKING OFF** (see **MASTURBATION**).

**JERKING OFF** (see **MASTURBATION**).

**JILLING OFF** (see **MASTURBATION**).

**KINSEY SCALE** A questionnaire in the form of a continuum that served to rate a person's attraction and behavior with regard to sex.

**KISSING** Touching lips with someone else's as an expression of love or desire.

**LABIA MAJORA** An outer layer of lips, which cover and protect the vagina.

**LABIA MINORA** An inner layer of lips, which cover and protect the vagina.

**LARC** Long-Acting, Reversible Contraception, which includes intra-uterine devices and contraceptive implants.

**LEGAL TRANSITION** Efforts to change one's identifying documentation to accurately reflect their gender identity.

**LESBIAN** A female who is attracted to another female.

**LUBRICATION** A substance designed or created to reduce friction.

**LUNELLE** A once-per-month birth control shot.

**MANUAL SEX** (see **MASTURBATION**).

**MASTURBATION** Sexual stimulation or rubbing (usually) of one's own genitals, to achieve sexual arousal—usually to the point of orgasm.

**MEDICAL TRANSITION** Undergoing physical procedures such as surgery or hormonal therapies to alter and match one's physical body to their internal experience.

**MENSTRUAL PRODUCTS** A range of devices and products to manage menstrual flow during one's period.

**MENSTRUATION** The shedding of the blood and membrane that would have formed the nourishing home in the uterus for an embryo to grow into a fetus (see **PERIOD**).

**METOIDIOPLASTY** A bottom surgery for FTM trans people in which the clitoris is released and made to appear longer that can allow for sexual sensation. This can sometimes be combined with a urethral extension to allow trans guys to pee while standing.

**MIFEPREX** (see **MIFEPRISTONE**).

**MIFEPRISTONE** Chemical abortion drug, which induces abortion in the first forty-nine days of gestation.

**MINORITY STRESS** The specific stress experienced by members of marginalized and stigmatized minority groups.

**MIRENA** (see **INTRAUTERINE SYSTEM**).

**MISSIONARY POSITION** A heterosexual sex position in which both partners face one another.

**MONOGAMY** Having sex with only one other person, within a committed long-term relationship.

**MONS** The fatty tissue above a woman's pubic bone—the part usually covered with hair.

**MORNING AFTER PILL** A misnomer for emergency contraception.

**NEGATIVE BODY IMAGE** A perception of ourselves that may not be true or that causes shame, anxiety, or self-consciousness.

**NOCTURNAL EMISSIONS** (see **WET DREAMS**).

**NOCTURNAL ORGASM** An orgasm experienced while asleep.

**NONOXYNOL-9** The most popular spermicide in America. It kills both sperm and HIV, but it also causes irritation to the internal vaginal and anal walls.

**NON-MARITAL SEX** Having sex without being married.

**NUVA-RING** (see **VAGINAL RING**).

**OBSTETRICS** The branch of the medical profession that deals with pregnancy and childbirth.

**OB/GYN** An initialism that stands for Obstetrics and Gynecology and/ or an Obstetrician/Gynecologist.

**ONE-NIGHT STAND** Sexual interactions that happen spontaneously between people who just met or do not know each other well (see **HOOKUP**).

**ORAL SEX** When one person puts their mouth or tongue on the genitals of another.

**ORGASM** The point at which sexual tension is released, creating waves of pleasurable sensations as well as muscular contractions of the penis (male) or vagina (female) and anus (both), which eventually end in intense feelings, often accompanied by ejaculation.

**ORIENTATION** What sex you choose to be sexual with and its relationship to your own (whether you are gay, straight, or bisexual).

**ORTHO-EVRA** (see **THE PATCH**).

**OUTERCOURSE** Sex with clothes on and/or that avoids penetration of any kind.

**OVARIES** Ovum- (or egg-) producing, reproductive organs in females.

**OVULATION** The release of the egg.

**PACKING** A method of social transition involving the placement of padding or prosthetics to create a more male-like crotch and curb dysphoria in FTM trans people.

**PASSING** A controversial term referring to being accepted as / believed to be in one's chosen gender without their trans status being known, discovered, or divulged.

**PASSING PRIVILEGE** The benefit and advantages a trans person may experience because their trans status is not known, discovered, or obvious.

**THE PATCH** A slow-releasing, hormonal patch, which prevents fertilization and implantation of eggs.

**PEGGING** A man being anally penetrated in some way by a female partner.

**PELVIC INFLAMMATORY DISEASE** (PID) A serious infection (usually the result of a sexually transmitted infection such as chlamydia or gonorrhea), which spreads from the vagina and cervix into the reproductive organ.

**PENIS** The reproductive organ, for male animals.

**PERIOD** (see **MENSTRUATION**).

**PERSONAL SAFETY** Things you can do ahead of time to keep yourself safe and lessen the chances of being victimized.

**PHYSICAL ABUSE** Shoving, hitting, choking, or anything that leaves bruises.

**PID** (see **PELVIC INFLAMMATORY DISEASE**).

**THE PILL** A pill of estrogen and/or progestin hormones, which is taken once a day to prevent the eggs from releasing, help thicken cervical mucus and/or prevent fertilized eggs from implanting in the uterus.

**PIV** Penis-In-Vagina sex.

**PLAN B** (see **EMERGENCY CONTRACEPTION**).

**PORNOGRAPHY** Media designed to sexually excite people.

**POSITIVE** (see **POZ**).

**POSITIVE BODY IMAGE** An acceptance of the unique qualities of our own bodies and a feeling of comfort and confidence with them.

**POST-EXPOSURE PROPHYLAZES** A month-long medication regimen, which greatly decreases the likelihood of HIV infection if taken within the first seventy-two hours of exposure.

**POZ** A term, particularly in the gay community, for people who are HIV-positive.

**POZ-SHAMING** Bullying or humiliating someone around their status as HIV-positive.

**PRE-CUM** Lubricating fluid released from the tip of a penis during arousal.

**PRE-EXPOSURE PROPHYLAXIS** An anti-HIV medication that keeps HIV-negative people from becoming infected. It is most commonly referred to by its prescription name, Truveda (see **PrEP**).

**PREGNANCY** The condition or duration of being pregnant.

**PREMARITAL SEX** A misnomer for sex prior to marriage. As marriage is not currently available to everyone, a more accurate term is non-marital sex.

**PREMATURE EJACULATION** Ejaculating very quickly or much more quickly than your partner.

**PREMENSTRUAL SYNDROME / PMS** A range of (typically negative) symptoms and effects that happen during the period between ovulation and menstruation.

**PREMENSTRUAL TENSION (PMT)** (see **PREMENSTRUAL SYNDROME**).

**PrEP** (see **PRE-EXPOSURE PROPHYLAXIS**).

**PRIDE** (A) The sense of satisfaction, community, and self-respect around the public display or acknowledgment of one's queerness. (B) Worldwide celebrations honoring the anniversary of the first public demonstrations for GLBT rights.

**PRIVILEGE** The benefit and advantages one gets because they belong to certain sets of the population. These sets include sex and gender, but also race, ethnicity, and socioeconomic status.

**PROSTATE GLAND** One of the glands that help create seminal fluid. The prostate is also called the "male G-Spot," and is considered a male erogenous zone.

**PUBERTY** The process that begins adolescence.

**PUBERTY BLOCKERS** A method of medical transition involving the prescription and use of medications that halt the puberty hormones that masculinize or feminize a body with secondary sex characteristics.

**PUBIC HAIR** Hair that grows on and around your genitals.

**PUBIC LICE** (see **CRABS**).

**PUSSY** (see **VAGINA**).

**QSA** (Queer Straight Alliance) Extracurricular, school-sponsored support and recreational club for queer youth and their allies (see **GSA**).

**QUEER** A sexual identity on the continuum other than straight.

**RAPE CULTURE** Judgments and cultural biases about women being targets of hostility, violence, or viewed as less-than, as property, or as only-there-for-sex.

**READ** (see **CLOCKED**).

**THE REAL-LIFE EXPERIENCE** A typically required period of (also typically) one year in which candidates for gender confirmation surgery live full-time as their true/preferred gender.

**THE REAL-LIFE TEST** (see **THE REAL-LIFE EXPERIENCE**).

**REFRACTORY PERIOD** The time between when someone has an orgasm before they can have another one.

**REPARATIVE THERAPY** Ineffective and harmful use of prayer, counseling, and sometimes drugs or shock therapy to "cure" gay people.

**RHYTHM METHODS** A natural contraceptive method which involves charting of the menstrual cycles in order to predict approximately nine "unsafe" days in which one does not have intercourse.

**RIMMING** (see **ANALINGUS**).

**RLE** (see **THE REAL-LIFE EXPERIENCE**).

**ROPHYS/ ROOFIES** Date rape drugs.

**RU-486** A previous name for Mifeprex/Mifepristone—a chemical abortion drug.

**SADDLEBACKING** Participating in oral and anal sex to mistakenly preserve virginity.

**SAFE SEX** A misnomer, which generally refers to abstinence, monogamy, or masturbation.

**SAFER SEX** Techniques that help reduce exposure to disease.

**SCABIES** (see **CRABS**).

**SCROTOPLASTY** A bottom surgery for FTM trans people in which the labia majora are used to form a scrotum.

**SCROTUM** The sac of skin and muscle that contains and (theoretically) protects the testicles.

**SEASONALE** A twelve-month regimen of birth control pills, which reduces periods to approximately four per year.

**SELF-ESTEEM** The ways in which one considers or feels about themselves as a person.

**SEMEN** The milky combination of sperm and other liquids gathered along the way. Also called "come" or "cum."

**SEX** One's physical parts and biological status as male or female.

**SEXTING** Sending graphic images and pornographic videos via text message to friends—considered child pornography if under eighteen.

**SEX TOY** A device designed for penetration of the vagina or anus, used by people of all genders and orientations for masturbation.

**SEXUAL ABUSE** Direct touching, fondling, and intercourse, against a person's will. Anything that takes away your ability to control how, where, or when you engage in sexual contact, including rape, unwanted touch, messing with your access to birth control, or repeatedly pressuring someone to have sex.

**SEXUAL ASSAULT** Unwanted sexual contact or threats, such as rape.

**SEXUAL EXPRESSION** What sex one chooses to be sexual with and its relationship to one's own. Sexual orientation refers to one's sexual attraction to men, women, both, or neither (see **SEXUAL ORIENTA-TION**).

**SEXUAL HARASSMENT** Unwelcome attention of a sexual nature.

**SEXUAL IDENTITY** Physical designation as male, female (or inter-sex) parts, based on hormones, chromosomes, and other body characteristics.

**SEXUAL ORIENTATION** What sex one chooses to be sexual with and its relationship to one's own. Sexual orientation refers to one's sexual attraction to men, women, both, or neither (see **SEXUAL EXPRESSION**).

**SEXUALLY TRANSMITTED DISEASES** Organisms, syndromes, and infections that are spread through sexual contact.

**SEXUALLY TRANSMITTED INFECTIONS** Organisms, syndromes, and infections that are spread through sexual contact.

**THE SHOT** An injection of hormones that prevent the releasing and joining of eggs as well as the implantation of fertilized eggs.

**SHOWER** A long, soft penis that does not increase much in length as it becomes erect.

**SITUATIONAL AWARENESS** Observing one's context and surroundings to assess the levels of safety and/or danger in one's environment.

**SLUT-SHAMING** Bullying or humiliating someone about the amount of sex someone has.

**SMEGMA** Bacteria, yeasts, stale urine, and dead skin cells that can collect under the foreskin of uncircumcised males to form a white, cheesy substance.

**SOCIAL TRANSITION** Behavioral steps made to culturally indicate one's gender identity and make others aware of it.

**SPERM** The male reproductive cells, comprised of twenty-three chromosomes, which (if joined by the DNA and chromosomes of an egg) create an embryo.

**SPERMICIDE** A foam, cream, jelly, film suppository or tablet placed inside the vagina, which kills and blocks sperm from entering the vaginal canal.

**THE SPONGE** A soft, disc-shaped device made of polyurethane foam, which contains spermicide, placed inside the vagina prior to sex.

**STDs** (see **SEXUALLY TRANSMITTED DISEASES**).

**STEALTH** (See **PASSING**).

**STEALTHING** A form of rape in which one person removes their condom without the other person's knowledge or consent.

**STEALTH-SHAMING** Behaviors stating, implying, or acting as though trans people who choose to not disclose their trans status are somehow not really trans.

**STERILIZATION** (see **VASECTOMY** or **TUBAL LIGATION**).

**STIs** (see **SEXUALLY TRANSMITTED INFECTIONS**).

**STRAIGHT** (see **HETEROSEXUAL**).

**STUFFING** A method of social transition involving using materials such as padding, bras, and prosthetic breasts to create cleavage and curb dysphoria in MTF trans people.

**SYPHILIS** A bacterial infection causing a series of symptoms including crater-like sores, a painful rash, and death.

**T CELLS** One specific type of blood cell that helps defend against infections and diseases.

**TESTICLES** Two small organs, which produce the male hormone (testosterone) and make sperm.

**TESTOSTERONE** The primary male hormone produced in the testicles.

**THEY** An alternative, gender-neutral pronoun to refer to a single person, instead of "he" or "she."

**TOP** The person penetrating someone else during anal sex.

**TOP SURGERY** A method of medical transition that involves either feminizing or masculinizing a trans person's torso.

**TOXIC SHOCK SYNDROME (TSS)** An infection associated with bacteria and toxins that can build up while using superabsorbent tampons.

**TRANSEXUAL** Alternative spelling of **TRANSSEXUAL** used to de-medicalize the term.

**TRANS-FETISHISM** Sexual attraction to a person's "transness" rather than the trans person themselves.

**TRANSGENDER** An umbrella term used to describe people whose gender identity (sense of themselves as male or female) or gender expression may differ from the parts they were born with.

**TRANSITION** The process of making changes to your appearance or biology, behavior, or legal status in order to live as a member of your true gender.

**TRANSSEXUAL** Out of date term to describe transgender people who have engaged in hormone therapies and/or surgical procedures.

**TRANSVESTITES** (Typically straight) people who wear the clothing of the opposite sex.

**TRICHOMONIASIS** A parasite, which causes irritation inside the penis, discharge with a strong odor, or a slight burning after urination and ejaculation.

**TROLL** A person who purposely causes trouble and harm through the Internet.

**TUBAL LIGATION** Surgically severing the tubes in which the sperm and egg meet in women to block pregnancy.

**TUCKING** A method of social transition involving hiding one's penis to create a more female-like crotch, and curb dysphoria in MTF trans people.

**URETHRA** The passage through the penis or vagina that opens to the outside to pass urine from the body.

**URETHRITIS** Inflammation caused by small amounts of bacteria or yeast in the vagina or urethra, which grow more than normal.

**URINARY TRACT INFECTION (UTI)** An infection caused by bacteria infecting the urethra or bladder.

**UTERUS** The womb in which the embryo attaches and eventually grows into a fetus.

**VAG/ VADGE** (see **VAGINA**).

**VAGINA** The reproductive organ for female mammals. It is also called a birth canal.

**VAGINAL RING** A combination of the pill and cervical cap in the form of a bendable, two-inch plastic ring worn around the cervix for three weeks each month.

**VAGINITIS** Inflammation caused by small amounts of bacteria or yeast in the vagina, which grow more than normal.

**VAGINOPLASTY** A bottom surgery for MTF trans people in which tissues of the scrotum and penis are used to fashion a largely functional vagina.

**VAS DEFERENS** The transport passageway of sperm to the urethra in males.

**VASECTOMY** Surgically severing the tubes that carry sperm in men to block pregnancy.

**VENEREAL DISEASES (VD)** (see **SEXUALLY TRANSMITTED DISEASES**).

**VERBAL ABUSE** Threats, insults, intimidation, isolation, or stalking (see **EMOTIONAL ABUSE**).

**VIBRATOR** A plastic, cylindrical wand that contains batteries and can be switched on to buzz pleasurably for masturbatory purposes.

**VIRGINITY** The state of sexual inexperience.

**WET DREAM** An orgasm experienced while asleep (often accompanied by an ejaculation for boys).

**WHATEVER-THE-PHOBIA** An umbrella term referring to an unclear or generalized fear of LGBT people and dynamics.

**WHORE** (see **SLUT**).

**WOODWORKING** (see **PASSING**).

**WPATH** The World Professional Association for Transgender Health responsible for outlined standards of care for people who are accessing medical transition.

**YEAST INFECTION** A fungal infection of the vagina.

**YOUTH-PRODUCED SEXUAL IMAGES** Sexualized pictures or texts created by minors.

# NOTES

## INTRO

1. "U.S. Teen Sexual Activity." Kaiser Family Foundation, 2005, accessed March 2016, http://enrichmentjournal.ag.org/200604/200604_4USTeenSex Acti.pdf.

2. Ibid.

3. "Internet Crimes Against Children." *Youth Internet Safety Survey*, 2001, accessed July 2016, http://www.ojp.usdoj.gov/ovc/publications/bulletins/inter net_2_2001/internet_2_01_6.html.

4. *"Sex and Tech: Results from a Survey of Teens and Young Adults."* The National Campaign to Prevent Teen and Unplanned Pregnancy, 2008, accessed December 2014, http://thenationalcampaign.org/resource/sex-and-tech.

5. "Child Sexual Abuse Statistics." The National Center for Victims of Crime, accessed November 2016, http://victimsofcrime.org/media/reporting-on -child-sexual-abuse/child-sexual-abuse-statistics.

6. Gary Remafedi, MD, MPH, James A. Farrow, MD, and Robert W. Deisher, MD. "Risk Factors for Attempted Suicide in Gay and Bisexual Youth." *Pediatrics* 87 (1991): 869–75.

7. "Famous LGBT People." Association for Lesbian Gay, Bisexual and Transgender Issues in Counseling, accessed October 2017, http://www.algbtical .org/2A%20PEOPLE.htm.

8. "Kevin Keller Receives Outstanding Comic Book at GLAAD Awards." GLAAD, 2013, accessed October 2017, https://www.glaad.org/tags/dan-parent.

9. *"Out* Magazine's Power 50 2017." *Out* Magazine, 2017, accessed October 2017, https://www.out.com/power-50/2017/7/19/power-50-2017.

10. *Your Guide to Understanding Genetic Conditions.* National Institutes of Health/US National Library of Medicine, accessed May 2016, https://ghr.nlm .nih.gov/chromosome/X.

## CHAPTER ONE

1. S. Dave, A. M. Johnson, K. A. Fenton, C. H. Mercer, B. Erens, and K. Wellings. "Male Circumcision in Britain: Findings from a National Probability Sample Survey." *Sexually Transmitted Infections* 79 (2003): 499–500.

## CHAPTER TWO

1. "Boys and Puberty." KidsHealth, accessed June 2011, http://kidshealth.org/kid/grow/boy/boys_puberty.html.
2. "Puberty." Planned Parenthood, accessed March 2015, https://www.plannedparenthood.org/learn/teens/puberty.
3. "Puberty." Planned Parenthood, accessed March 2015, https://www.plannedparenthood.org/learn/teens/puberty.

## CHAPTER THREE

1. "Puberty." Planned Parenthood, accessed March 2015, https://www.plannedparenthood.org/learn/teens/puberty.
2. Jo Langford, *Spare Me 'The Talk!'* (Seattle: ParentMap, 2016), 8.
3. "Toxic Shock Syndrome." The Mayo Clinic, accessed October 2015, http://www.mayoclinic.org/diseases-conditions/toxic-shock-syndrome/basics/definition/con-20021326.
4. Todd Nivin, MD, reviewer. "Menstrual Blood Problems." WebMD, September 29, 2014, accessed October 2015, http://www.webmd.com/women/guide/menstrual-blood-problems-clots-color-and-thickness.
5. Barcligt Songhai, MD. "Premenstrual Syndrome (PMS) Fact Sheet." 2010, Office of Women's Health, accessed July 2011, http://www.womenshealth.gov/publications/our-publications/fact-sheet/premenstrual-syndrome.html.
6. Jo Langford. *Spare Me 'The Talk!'* (Seattle: ParentMap, 2016), 11.
7. Jessica Kane. "Here's How Much A Woman's Period Will Cost Her Over A Lifetime." Huffington Post, May 18, 2015, accessed October 2015, http://www.huffingtonpost.com/2015/05/18/period-cost-lifetime_n_7258780.html.
8. B. H. Cottrell. "An Updated Review of Evidence to Discourage Douching." *MCN, The American Journal of Maternal Child Nursing* 35 (2) (March–April 2010): 102–7; quiz 108–9.
9. "Breast Implants Linked with Suicide." Reuters, last modified August 9, 2007, accessed November 2015, http://www.reuters.com/article/us-implants-suicide-idUSN0836919020070809.

10. "Breast Self-Exams." Johns Hopkins Medical Center, Breast Center, accessed November 2015, http://www.hopkinsmedicine.org/breast_center/treatments_services/breast_cancer_screening/breast_self_exam.html.

11. "Symptoms and Signs." National Breast Cancer Foundation, accessed November 2015, http://www.nationalbreastcancer.org/breast-cancer-symptoms-and-signs.

12. "The Initial Reproductive Health Visit." American College of Obstetricians and Gynecologists, Committee on Adolescent Health, Opinion No. 460. *Obstetrics and Gynecology* 2010: 240–43.

## CHAPTER FOUR

1. Debby Herbenick, PhD, MPH. "Erect Penile Length and Circumference Dimensions of 1,661 Sexually Active Men in the United States." *Journal of Sexual Medicine* 11 (January 2014): 93–101. Article first published online: July 10, 2013.

2. David Veale, Sarah Miles, Sally Bramley, Gordon Muir, and John Hodsoll. "Am I Normal? A Systematic Review and Construction of Nomograms for Flaccid and Erect Penis Length and Circumference in Up to 15,521 Men." *BJU International.* Wiley Online Library, accessed September 2015, http://onlinelibrary.wiley.com/doi/10.1111/bju.13010/full.

3. "How the Penis Works." WebMD, accessed October 2017, https://www.webmd.com/erectile-dysfunction/how-an-erection-occurs.

4. "Pelvic Floor Anatomy and Applied Physiology." National Institutes of Health, September 2009, accessed October 2017, https://www.ncbi.nlm.nih.gov/pmc/articles/PMC2617789/.

## CHAPTER FIVE

1. Jo Langford. *Spare Me 'The Talk!'* (Seattle: ParentMap, 2016), 20.

2. "Gender Dysphoria." DSM5.org, American Psychiatric Association, 2013, accessed June 2016, http://www.dsm5.org/documents-Gender-Dysphoria.pdf.

3. Ibid.

4. "Eating Disorder Statistics." South Carolina Department of Mental Health, 2006, accessed February 2011, http://www.state.sc.us/dmh/anorexia/statistics.htm.

5. Ibid.

6. Jo Langford. *Spare Me 'The Talk!'* (Seattle: ParentMap, 2015), 14.

7. Ibid. Accessed May 2011.

## CHAPTER SIX

1. Jo Langford. *Spare Me 'The Talk!'* (Seattle: ParentMap, 2016), 23.
2. Ibid., 23–24.
3. Gary Gates. "How Many Adults Identify as Transgender in the United States." The Williams Institute, accessed July 2016, http://williamsinstitute.law.ucla.edu/research/how-many-adults-identify-as-transgender-in-the-united-states.
4. "Small Share of Americans in Active Military Duty." Pew Research, May 2012, accessed July 2016, http://www.pewresearch.org/daily-number/small-share-of-americans-in-active-military-duty.
5. GLAAD Media Reference Guide—In Focus: Covering the Transgender Community. https://www.glaad.org/reference/covering-trans-community.

## CHAPTER SEVEN

1. Jo Langford. *Spare Me 'The Talk!'* (Seattle: ParentMap, 2016), 25.
2. "1,500 Animal Species Practice Homosexuality." *News Medical*, 2006, accessed September 2016, http://www.news-medical.net/news/2006/10/23/1500-animal-species-practice-homosexuality.aspx.
3. Gary J. Gates. "How Many People Are Lesbian, Gay, Bisexual and Transgender?" The Williams Institute at UCLA School of Law, April 2011, accessed April 2011, http://williamsinstitute.law.ucla.edu/research/census-lgbt-demographics-studies/how-many-people-are-lesbian-gay-bisexual-and-transgender.
4. Kinsey's Heterosexual-Homosexual Rating Scale. The Kinsey Institute, 2009, accessed September 2011, http://www.iub.edu/~kinsey/research/ak-hhscale.html.
5. Anthony Bogaert. "Exactly What Percentage of the World's Population Is Asexual?" Queerty.com, accessed July 2016, http://www.queerty.com/exactly-what-percentage-of-the-worlds-population-is-asexual-20150727.
6. Ibid.

## PART THREE

1. B. A. Robinson. "Reparative Therapy: Statements by Professional Associations and Their Leaders." Religious Tolerance, 2006, accessed June 2011, http://religioustolerance.org/hom_prof3.htm.
2. "Homosexual Behavior Due to Genetics and Environmental Factors." Biology News Net, 2008, accessed June 2011, http://www.biologynews.net/

archives/2008/06/29/homosexual_behavior_due_to_genetics_and_environmen tal_factors.html.

## CHAPTER EIGHT

1. Jo Langford. *Spare Me 'The Talk!'* (Seattle: ParentMap, 2016), 28.
2. Ibid., 30.
3. Gary Remafedi, MD, MPH, James A. Farrow, MD, and Robert W. Deisher, MD. "Risk Factors for Attempted Suicide in Gay and Bisexual Youth." *Pediatrics* 87 (1991): 869–75.
4. R. L. Spitzer. "The Diagnostic Status of Homosexuality in DSM-III: A Reformulation of the Issues." *American Journal of Psychiatry* 138 (1981): 210–15.
5. "Matthew Shepard and James Byrd, Jr. Hate Crimes Prevention Act." Human Rights Campaign, last modified February 1, 2010, accessed November 2011, http://www.hrc.org/resources/entry/questions-and-answers-the-matthew -shepard-and-james-byrd-jr.-hate-crimes-pr.
6. "Sexual Conversion? American Psychological Association Says Not Through Psychotherapy." PsychiatricTimes.com, accessed August 2011, http:// www.psychiatrictimes.com/articles/sexual-"conversion"-american-psychological -association-says-not-through-psychotherapy.

## CHAPTER NINE

1. "A Survey of LGBT Americans." Pew Research Center, accessed June 2016, http://www.pewsocialtrends.org/2013/06/13/a-survey-of-lgbt-americans.

## CHAPTER ELEVEN

1. "Tips for Allies of Transgender People." GLAAD, accessed April 2014, http://www.glaad.org/transgender/allies.
2. "10 Steps for Starting a GSA." GSA Network, accessed August 2016, https://gsanetwork.org/resources/building-your-gsa/10-steps-starting-gsa.

## CHAPTER TWELVE

1. Johnson, Ramon. "Gay Population Statistics." Liveabout.com, accessed June 2016, https://www.liveabout.com/gay-population-statistics-in-the-united -states-1410784.

2. *Standards of Care for the Health of Transsexual, Transgender, and Gender Nonconforming People, Seventh Version* (PDF). World Professional Association for Transgender Health, accessed July 2016, http://www.wpath.org/site_page .cfm?pk_association_webpage_menu=1351&pk_association_webpage=3926.

3. Norman P. Spack, Laura Edwards-Leeper, Henry A. Feldman, Scott Leibowitz, Francie Mandel, David A. Diamond, and Stanley R. Vance. "Children and Adolescents with Gender Identity Disorder Referred to a Pediatric Medical Center." *Journal of Pediatrics*, accessed August 2016, http://pediatrics.aappublications.org/content/129/3/418.

4. Wylie C. Hembree, Peggy Cohen-Kettenis, Henriette A. Delemarre-van de Waal, Louis J. Gooren, Walter J. Meyer III, Norman P. Spack, Vin Tangpricha, and Victor M. Montori. "Endocrine Treatment of Transsexual Persons: An Endocrine Society Clinical Practice Guideline." Accessed June 2016, https:// academic.oup.com/jcem/article/94/9/3132/2596324/Endocrine-Treatment-of -Transsexual-Persons-An.

5. Mitch Kellway. "Blocking Puberty Is Beneficial for Transgender Youth." Advocate.com, accessed June 2016, http://www.advocate.com/politics/transgen der/2014/09/14/study-blocking-puberty-beneficial-transgender-youth.

6. "Information on Transitioning and Transgender Health." RevelandRiot. com, accessed June 2016, http://www.revelandriot.com/resources/trans-health/.

7. Ibid.

8. Ibid.

9. Ibid.

10. Masculinising Hormone Information. Gendercentre.org, accessed July 2016, https://gendercentre.org.au/images/Services/Female_to_Male/Masculini sing_Hormone_Information.pdf.

11. Feminising Hormone Information. Gendercentre.org, accessed July 2016.

12. E. Coleman et al. "Standards of Care for the Health of Transsexual, Transgender, and Gender-Nonconforming People." *International Journal of Transgenderism* 13(4), 165–232, accessed February 2016, doi:10.1080/15532739. 2011.

13. Ejeris Dixon, Chai Jindasurat, and Victor Tobar. "Hate Violence Against Lesbian, Gay, Bisexual, Transgender, Queer and HIV-Affected Communities." AVP.org. National Coalition of Anti-Violence Programs, accessed July 2016, https://avp.org/wp-content/uploads/2017/04/2011_NCAVP_HV_Reports.pdf.

14. *Standards of Care for the Health of Transsexual, Transgender, and Gender Nonconforming People, Seventh Version* (PDF). World Professional Association for Transgender Health, accessed July 2016, http://www.wpath.org/site_page .cfm?pk_association_webpage_menu=1351&pk_association_webpage=3926.

15. Ibid.

16. Gender Transition Applicants. US Department of State, accessed July 2016, https://travel.state.gov/content/passports/en/passports/information/gender.html.

17. Social Security Administration Updates Gender Change Policy. TransgenderLawCenter.org, accessed June 2016, http://transgenderlawcenter.org/archives/8339.

18. FAQ About Identity Documents. Lambda Legal, accessed July 2016, http://www.lambdalegal.org/know-your-rights/transgender/identity-document-faq#Q4.

19. Know Your Rights/Passports. TransEquality.org, accessed July 2016, http://www.transequality.org/know-your-rights/passports.

## CHAPTER FOURTEEN

1. "Accelerating Acceptance." GLAAD, accessed July 2017, http://www.glaad.org/files/2016_GLAAD_Accelerating_Acceptance.pdf.

## CHAPTER FIFTEEN

1. Patrick Fagan and Robert Rector. "The Effects of Divorce on America." Heritage.org, accessed July 2016, http://www.heritage.org/research/reports/2000/06/the-effects-of-divorce-on-america.

## CHAPTER SIXTEEN

1. Jo Langford. *Spare Me 'The Talk!'* (Seattle: ParentMap, 2016), 40, 41.

2. Ibid., 43.

3. "Teen Dating Violence Among LGBTQ Youth." Human Rights Campaign, HRC.org, accessed July 2016, http://www.hrc.org/resources/teen-dating-violence-among-lgbtq-youth.

4. CDC Morbidity and Mortality Weekly Report. "Sexual Identity, Sex of Sexual Contacts, and Health-Related Behaviors Among Students in Grades 9–12—United States and Selected Sites, 2015." Centers for Disease Control and Prevention, CDC.org, accessed August 2016, https://www.cdc.gov/mmwr/volumes/65/ss/ss6509a1.html.

5. Ibid.

6. Jo Langford. *Spare Me 'The Talk!'* (Seattle: ParentMap, 2016), 44.

7. Ibid.

## CHAPTER SEVENTEEN

1. Franklin Lowe, MD, MPH, FACS. "All About Semen." Menstuff, 2006, accessed July 2011, http://www.menstuff.org/issues/byissue/semen.html.

2. Dan Savage. "Savage Love: Play with Her Clit." *The Stranger*, July 19, 2007.

3. Jo Langford. *Spare Me 'The Talk!'* (Seattle: ParentMap, 2016), 48.

4. "Alice" (a team of Columbia University health educators, health care providers, other health professionals, and information and research specialists and writers). "Masturbation Healthy?" *Go Ask Alice!* Columbia University, accessed February 2011, http://www.goaskalice.columbia.edu/answered-questions/masturbation-healthy.

5. M. Gerressu, C. H. Mercer, C. A. Graham, K. Wellings, and A. M. Johnson. "Prevalence of Masturbation and Associated Factors in a British National Probability Survey." *Archives of Sexual Behavior* 37 (2) (April 2008): 266–78.

6. Jerry Ropelato. "Internet Pornography Statistics." Top Ten Reviews, 2006, accessed August 2011, http://internet-filter-review.toptenreviews.com/internet-pornography-statistics.html.

7. Onur Güntürkün. "Adult Persistence of Head-Turning Asymmetry." *Nature* (February 13, 2003), 421, 711.

8. Jo Langford. *Spare Me 'The Talk!'* (Seattle: ParentMap, 2016), 58.

9. Ibid.

10. Ibid.

11. Dan Savage. "Savage Love: Wiggle Room." *The Stranger*, February 25, 2010.

12. Em & Lo. "The Bottom Line." *New York* Magazine, October 25, 2007.

13. Jo Langford. *Spare Me 'The Talk!'* (Seattle: ParentMap, 2016), 61.

14. "HIV Transmission." Centers for Disease Control and Prevention, accessed March 2011, https://www.cdc.gov/hiv/basics/prevention.html.

15. William Saletan. "Ass Backwards: The Media's Silence About Rampant Anal Sex." Slate, posted September 20, 2005, http://www.slate.com/id/2126643.

16. Jo Langford. *Spare Me 'The Talk!'* (Seattle: ParentMap, 2016), 62–63.

## CHAPTER EIGHTEEN

1. Jo Langford. *Spare Me 'The Talk!'* (Seattle: ParentMap, 2016), 65.

## CHAPTER NINETEEN

1. Jo Langford. *Spare Me 'The Talk!'* (Seattle: ParentMap, 2016), 68, 69.

# CHAPTER TWENTY

1. "Sexually Transmitted Diseases (STDs)." Planned Parenthood, 2011, accessed June 2011, http://www.plannedparenthood.org/health-topics/stds-hiv -safer-sex-101.htm.

2. Jo Langford. *Spare Me 'The Talk!'* (Seattle: ParentMap, 2016), 72–78.

3. Vanessa Cullins, MD. "Chlamydia." Planned Parenthood, updated 2011, accessed June 2011, http://www.plannedparenthood.org/health-info/stds-hiv -safer-sex/chlamydia.

4. "Reported Cases of Sexually Transmitted Diseases on the Rise, Some at Alarming Rate." NCHHSTP Newsroom, Centers for Disease Control and Prevention, November 17, 2015, accessed November 2015, http://www.cdc.gov/ nchhstp/newsroom/2015/std-surveillance-report-press-release.html.

5. Ibid.

6. Ibid.

7. "Genital Herpes Statistics." Herpes Clinic, accessed March 2016, http:// www.herpesclinic.com/genitalherpes/genitalherpesstatistics/.

8. "The ABCs of Viral Hepatitis." Centers for Disease Control and Prevention, 2011, accessed August 2011, http://www.cdc.gov/Features/ViralHep atitis.

9. Ibid.

10. "Hepatitis B Vaccine (Recombinant)." Merck and Co. Inc., 2011, accessed July 2011, http://www.merck.com/product/usa/pi_circulars/r/recombivax_hb/ recombivax_pi.pdf.

11. Harvey Simon, MD. "Hepatitis B." *New York Times*, accessed September 2011, http://health.nytimes.com/health/guides/disease/rubella/hepatitis-b.html.

12. "Hepatitis B Foundation Participates in U.S. Capitol Briefing." Hepatitis B Foundation, 2005, accessed July 2011, http://www.hepb.org/pdf/Capi tol_Briefing7_05.pdf.

13. "Information About Gardasil." Gardasil.com, accessed August 2011, http:// www.gardasil.com.

14. "Study: Half of Men May Be Infected with HPV." Huffington Post, 2011, accessed March 2011, http://www.huffingtonpost.com/2011/02/28/half -men-infected-hpv_n_829449.html.

15. "STD Awareness Month Facts." Minnesota Department of Health, 2011, accessed April 2011, http://www.health.state.mn.us/divs/idepc/dtopics/stds/ stdbasics.html.

16. "STDs in America: How Many Cases and at What Cost?" American Social Health Association/Kaiser Family Foundation, 1998, accessed March 2016, http://kff.org/hivaids/sexually-transmitted-diseases-in-america-how-many/.

17. "11 Facts About Teens and STIS." DoSomething.org, accessed June 2011, http://www.dosomething.org/tipsandtools/11-facts-about-teens-and-stds.

18. "STDs in Adolescents and Young Adults." Centers for Disease Control and Prevention, 2010, accessed December 2010, http://www.cdc.gov/std/stats09/adol.htm.

## CHAPTER TWENTY-ONE

1. Jo Langford. *Spare Me 'The Talk!'* (Seattle: ParentMap, 2016), 80–83.

2. Sarah Childress. "CDC Reports Troubling Rise in HIV Infections Among Young People." PBS.org, accessed July 2016, http://www.pbs.org/wgbh/front line/article/cdc-reports-troubling-rise-in-hiv-infections-among-young-people/.

3. "Condoms and STDs." Centers for Disease Control and Prevention, 2014, accessed December 2014, http://www.cdc.gov/condomeffectiveness/docs/con doms_and_stds.pdf.

4. Truvada website, http://www.truvada.com.

5. Rod McCullom. "Lowering the Age for HIV Prevention." *The Atlantic*, February 11, 2015, accessed November 2015, http://www.theatlantic.com/health/archive/2015/02/lowering-the-age-for-hiv-prevention/385303/.

6. R. M. Grant, J. R. Lama, P. L. Anderson, et al.: iPrEx Study Team. "Preexposure Chemoprophylaxis for HIV Prevention in Men Who Have Sex with Men." *New England Journal of Medicine* 363 (27) (2010): 2587–99, accessed November 2015, http://www.nejm.org/doi/full/10.1056/NEJMoa1011205.

7. "Preventing Sexual Transmission of HIV." AIDS.gov, accessed November 2016, https://www.hiv.gov/hiv-basics/hiv-prevention/reducing-sexual-risk/preventing-sexual-transmission-of-hiv.

8. "HIV Among Youth." Centers for Disease Control and Prevention, April 27, 2016 (accessed July 2016), http://www.cdc.gov/hiv/group/age/youth/.

9. "Doppelgangland." *Buffy The Vampire Slayer*. Writ. Joss Whedon, Dir. Joss Whedon, Fox, 1999.

## CHAPTER TWENTY-TWO

1. Heather Boonstra. "Condoms, Contraceptives and Nonoxynol-9: Complex Issues Obscured by Ideology." *Guttmacher Report on Public Policy* 8 (2) (May 2005): 4–6, 16.

2. Jo Langford. *Spare Me 'The Talk!'* (Seattle: ParentMap, 2016), 89–90.

3. R. G. Frezieres, T. L. Walsh, A. L. Nelson, V. A. Clark, and A. H. Coulson. "Breakage and Acceptability of a Polyurethane Condom: A Randomized,

Controlled Study." National Library of Medicine / National Institutes of Health, accessed February 2015, https://www.ncbi.nlm.nih.gov/pubmed/9561872.

4. K. Davis, C. A. Stappenbeck, J. Norris, W. H. George, A. J. Jacques-Tiura, T. J. Schraufnagel, and K. F. Kajumulo. "Young Men's Condom Use Resistance Tactics: A Latent Profile Analysis." *Journal of Sex Research* 51 (4).

5. A. Zibners, B. A. Cromer, and J. Hayes. "Comparison of Continuation Rates for Hormonal Contraception Among Adolescents." *Journal of Pediatric and Adolescent Gynecology* 12 (1999): 90–94, http://www.ncbi.nlm.nih.gov/pubmed/10326194.

6. T. R. Raine, A. Foster-Rosales, U. D. Upadhyay, et al. "One-Year Contraceptive Continuation and Pregnancy in Adolescent Girls and Women Initiating Hormonal Contraceptives." *Obstetrics & Gynecology* 117 (February 2011): 363–71, accessed February 2015, http://www.ncbi.nlm.nih.gov/pubmed/21252751.

7. "Plan B: The New Morning After Pill." Estronaut, A Forum for Women's Health, accessed 2011, http://www.estronaut.com/a/Plan_B_Morning_After_Emergency_Contraceptive.htm.

## CHAPTER TWENTY-THREE

1. Jo Langford. *Spare Me 'The Talk!'* (Seattle: ParentMap, 2016), 101–4.
2. Ibid., 101.
3. Ibid., 53.

## CHAPTER TWENTY-FOUR

1. Mark Potok. "Anti-Gay Hate Crimes: Doing the Math." SPLawCenter.org, accessed July 2017, https://www.splcenter.org/fighting-hate/intelligence-report/2011/anti-gay-hate-crimes-doing-math.

## CHAPTER TWENTY-FIVE

1. Jo Langford. *Spare Me 'The Talk!'* (Seattle: ParentMap, 2016), 107.
2. Carla Van Dam, PhD. *Identifying Child Molesters* (New York: Haworth Maltreatment and Trauma Press, 2001), 50.
3. Wendy Maltz. *The Sexual Healing Journey: A Guide for Survivors of Sexual Abuse* (New York: HarperCollins, 2001), 30.
4. Jo Langford. *Spare Me 'The Talk!'* (Seattle: ParentMap, 2016), 108–9.
5. "Key Facts." National Center for Missing and Exploited Children, 2009, accessed August 2015, http://www.missingkids.com/KeyFacts.

6. Howard Snyder. *Sexual Assault of Young Children as Reported to Law Enforcement: Victim, Incident, and Offender Characteristics*: "Table 1: Age Profile of the Victims of Sexual Assault." US Department of Justice, Bureau of Justice Statistics, accessed June 2016, https://www.bjs.gov/content/pub/pdf/saycrle.pdf.

7. Michelle Lynberg Black, PhD, MPH. "The National Intimate Partner and Sexual Violence Survey." Centers for Disease Control and Prevention, National Center for Injury Prevention and Control, Division of Violence Prevention, accessed December 2015, http://vawnet.org/Assoc_Files_VAWnet/NRCWebinar_NISVSBriefingHandout.pdf.

8. Jo Langford. *Spare Me 'The Talk!'* (Seattle: ParentMap, 2016), 110–11.

9. Ibid., 115.

10. Susan Weiss. "Date Rape Drugs Fact Sheet." Department of Health and Human Services Office on Women's Health, accessed August 2011, http://womenshealth.gov/publications/our-publications/fact-sheet/date-rape-drugs.html.

11. Mary Koss and Mary Harvey. *The Rape Victim: Clinical and Community Interventions* (Newbury Park, CA: Sage Library of Social Research, 1991).

## CHAPTER TWENTY-SIX

1. "Statistics." RAINN.org, accessed March 2016, https://rainn.org/statistics.

2. "U.S. Departments of Justice and Education Release Joint Guidance to Help Schools Ensure the Civil Rights of Transgender Students." Department of Justice, accessed May 2016, https://www.justice.gov/opa/pr/us-departments-justice-and-education-release-joint-guidance-help-schools-ensure-civil-rights.

3. Ibid.

4. Alla Dastagir. "The Imaginary Predator in America's Transgender Bathroom War." USAToday.com, accessed June 2016, http://www.usatoday.com/story/news/nation/2016/04/28/transgender-bathroom-bills-discrimination/32594395.

## CHAPTER TWENTY-SEVEN

1. Peter Fields. "The Truth About Homophobia." HuffingtonPost.com, accessed October 2017, https://www.huffingtonpost.com/entry/the-truth-about-homophobia_us_57ae12aee4b0ae60ff026207.

2. William Grimes. "George Weinberg Dies at 87; Coined 'Homophobia' After Seeing Fear of Gays." The *New York Times*, accessed October 2017, https://www.nytimes.com/2017/03/22/us/george-weinberg-dead-coined-homophobia.html.

3. Odium. *Oxford English Dictionary*. Accessed October 2017, https://en.oxforddictionaries.com/definition/odium.

# CHAPTER TWENTY-EIGHT

1. Michael Dentato. "The Minority Stress Perspective." American Psychological Association, accessed June 2016, http://www.apa.org/pi/aids/resources/exchange/2012/04/minority-stress.aspx.

2. "Statistics You Should Know About Gay & Transgender Students." PFLAG.org, accessed June 2016, http://www.pflagnyc.org/safeschools/statistics.

3. Jerome Hunt. "Why the Gay and Transgender Population Experiences Higher Rates of Substance Use." Center for American Progress, accessed June 2016, https://www.americanprogress.org/issues/lgbt/report/2012/03/09/11228/why-the-gay-and-transgender-population-experiences-higher-rates-of-substance-use.

4. Zack Ford. "STUDY: 40 Percent of Homeless Youth Are LGBT, Family Rejection Is Leading Cause." Thinkprogress.org, accessed July 2016, https://thinkprogress.org/study-40-percent-of-homeless-youth-are-lgbt-family-rejection-is-leading-cause-a2aaa72c414a/.

5. Lila Shapiro. "New Report Offers a Look at 'Survival Sex' and the LGBTQ Youth Who Are Turning to It." Huffington Post, accessed June 2016, http://www.huffingtonpost.com/2015/02/26/lgbt-homeless-youth-survival-sex_n_6754248.html.

6. "Suicide Facts." Suicide Prevention Education for Kids, accessed January 2016, http://www.speakforthem.org/facts.html.

7. "How Do Mental Health Conditions Affect the LGBTQ Community?" National Alliance on Mental Health Issues, accessed May 2016, http://www.nami.org/Find-Support/LGBTQ.

8. "Sexual Identity, Sex of Sexual Contacts, and Health-Risk Behaviors Among Students in Grades 9–12: Youth Risk Behavior Surveillance." US Department of Health and Human Services, Centers for Disease Control and Prevention, accessed June 2013, https://www.researchgate.net/publication/281044134_Sexual_identity_sex_of_sexual_contacts_and_health-risk_behaviors_among_students_in_grades_9-12-Youth_Risk_Behavior_Surveillance_selected_sites_United_States.

9. I. H. Meyer and M. E. Northridge (Eds.). *The Health of Sexual Minorities: Public Health Perspectives on Lesbian, Gay, Bisexual and Transgender Populations* (New York: Springer, 2007).

10. Jessica F. Morris, Craig R. Waldo, and Esther D. Rothblum. "A Model of Predictors and Outcomes of Outness Among Lesbian and Bisexual Women." *American Journal of Orthopsychiatry, Mental Health and Social Justice*, accessed May 2016, http://onlinelibrary.wiley.com/doi/10.1037/0002-9432.71.1.61/abstract.

11. Scott L. Hershberger and Anthony R. D'Augelli. "The Impact of Victimization on the Mental Health and Suicidality of Lesbian, Gay, and Bisexual Youths." *Developmental Psychology* 31 (1), January 1995.

12. Ilan Meyer. "Prejudice, Social Stress, and Mental Health in Lesbian, Gay, and Bisexual Populations: Conceptual Issues and Research Evidence." National Institutes of Health, accessed June 2016, https://www.ncbi.nlm.nih.gov/pmc/articles/PMC2072932/.

13. TabooJive. "Stonewall: Freedom Overdue." Stop-Homophobia.com, accessed June 2016, http://www.stop-homophobia.com/thestonewallriots.htm.

14. "Stonewall Riots: The Beginning of the LGBT Movement." The Leadership Conference, accessed June 2016, https://greenwichvillagehistory.wordpress.com/tag/stonewall/.

## CHAPTER TWENTY-NINE

1. Jeremy Gibbs. "Religious Conflict, Sexual Identity, and Suicidal Behaviors Among LGBT Young Adults." US National Library of Medicine / National Institutes of Health. March 2015 (accessed June 2016), https://www.ncbi.nlm.nih.gov/pubmed/25763926.

2. Ibid.

3. Rodrigues Pereira. "Internalized Homophobia and Suicidal ideation Among LGBT Youth." *Journal of Psychiatry*, accessed June 2016, http://www.omicsonline.com/open-access/internalized-homophobia-and-suicidal-ideation-among-lgb-youth-Psychiatry-1000229.php?aid=41252.

## CHAPTER THIRTY

1. Zack Ford. "STUDY: 40 Percent Of Homeless Youth Are LGBT, Family Rejection Is Leading Cause." Thinkprogress.org, accessed July 2016, https://thinkprogress.org/study-40-percent-of-homeless-youth-are-lgbt-family-rejection-is-leading-cause-a2aaa72c414a/.

## CHAPTER THIRTY-ONE

1. "Youth Internet Safety Survey." *Internet Crimes Against Children*, accessed July 2011, http://www.ojp.usdoj.gov/ovc/publications/bulletins/internet_2_2001/internet_2_01_6.html.

2. Ibid.

3. Ibid.

4. Gavin De Becker. *The Gift of Fear* (New York: Dell Publishing, 1997).

5. Heather J. Clawson, Nicole Dutch, Amy Solomon, and Lisa Goldblatt-Grace. "Human Trafficking Into and Within the United States: A Review of the Literature." Office of the Assistant Secretary for Planning and Evaluation, US Department of Health and Social Services, accessed November 2015, http://aspe.hhs.gov/basic-report/human-trafficking-and-within-united-states-review-literature.

6. Kevin Bales. "The Number." The CNN Freedom Project: Ending Modern Day Slavery, accessed November 2015, http://thecnnfreedomproject.blogs.cnn.com/category/the-facts/the-number.

7. Clawson, Dutch, Solomon, and Goldblatt-Grace. "Human Trafficking Into and Within the United States."

8. Clawson, Dutch, Solomon, and Goldblatt-Grace. "Human Trafficking Into and Within the United States."

## CHAPTER THIRTY-TWO

1. Bev Betkowski. "Rural Teen Boys Most Likely to Access Pornography, Study Shows." Faculty News, University of Alberta, accessed March 2016, www.eurekalert.org/pub_releases/2007-02/uoa-oit022307.php.

2. "Online Safety Statistics." My Internet Safety Coach, accessed December 2010, http://myinternetsafetycoach.com/?p=18.

3. Jerry Ropelato. "Internet Pornography Statistics." Top Ten Reviews, 2006, accessed August 2011, http://internet-filter-review.toptenreviews.com/internet-pornography-statistics.html.

## CHAPTER THIRTY-THREE

1. "Social Media and Kids: Some Benefits, Some Worries." The American Academy of Pediatrics, accessed May 2015, https://www.aap.org/en-us/about-the-aap/aap-press-room/pages/Social-Media-and-Kids-Some-Benefits,-Some-Worries.aspx.

2. Jo Langford. Spare Me 'The Talk!' (Seattle: ParentMap, 2016), 126–29.

3. Murad Ahmed. "Teen 'Sexting' Craze Leading to Child Porn Arrests in U.S." The Times (London), January 2017, https://www.thetimes.co.uk/article/teen-sexting-craze-leading-to-child-porn-arrests-in-us-2tlhkgmtqsr.

4. Jo Langford. Spare Me 'The Talk!' (Seattle: ParentMap, 2016), 130.

5. "Sexual Offenses: Federal Law 18 U.S.C. 1466A—Obscene Visual Representations of the Sexual Abuse of Children." SexLaws.org, accessed March 2016, https://www.law.cornell.edu/uscode/text/18/1466A.

6. Jo Langford. *Spare Me 'The Talk!'* (Seattle: ParentMap, 2016), 133–37.

7. "Cyberbullying." *Trends & Tudes*, April 2007 (Vol. 6, issue 4), Harris Interactive, http://www.ncpc.org/resources/files/pdf/bullying/Cyberbullying%20Trends%20-%20Tudes.pdf.

8. "Teens, Kindness and Cruelty on Social Network Sites." Pew Research Center, Family Online Safety Institute, Cable in the Classroom, accessed November 9, 2011, http://www.pewinternet.org/2011/11/09/teens-kindness-and-cruelty-on-social-network-sites-2.

9. "Teen Online and Wireless Safety Survey: Cyberbullying, Sexting and Parental Controls." Cox Communications, in partnership with the National Center for Missing and Exploited Children, accessed May 2009, http://www.cox.com/wcm/en/aboutus/datasheet/takecharge/2009-teen-survey.pdf.

10. Roy Benaroch, MD. "Preventing Teen Suicide." WebMD.com, February 3, 2012, http://teens.webmd.com/preventing-teen-suicide.

11. Mitch Van Geel, PhD, Paul Vedder, PhD, and Jenny Tanilon, PhD. "Relationship Between Peer Victimization, Cyberbullying, and Suicide in Children and Adolescents: A Meta-Analysis." *JAMA Pediatrics* 168 (5): 435–42. Published online March 10, 2014, http://www.ncbi.nlm.nih.gov/pubmed/24615300.

# CHAPTER THIRTY-FOUR

1. Carol Lee. "Gay Teens Ignored by High School Sex Ed Classes." Women's eNews, accessed February 2017, http://womensenews.org/2002/02/gay-teens-ignored-high-school-sex-ed-classes.

2. Brendan McDermon. The Power of Inclusive Sex-Ed. *The Atlantic*, accessed October 2017, https://www.theatlantic.com/education/archive/2017/07/the-power-of-inclusive-sex-ed/533772/

3. "Sex and HIV Education." Guttmacher.org, accessed May 2016, https://www.guttmacher.org/state-policy/explore/sex-and-hiv-education.

4. "HIV Among Youth." Centers for Disease Control and Prevention, accessed April 27, 2016, http://www.cdc.gov/hiv/group/age/youth/index.html.

5. "Syphilis & MSM (Men Who Have Sex With Men)—CDC Fact Sheet." Centers for Disease Control and Prevention, accessed April 27, 2016, http://www.cdc.gov/std/Syphilis/STDFact-MSM-Syphilis.htm.

6. "New Study Finds HIV Risk Among Sexual-Minority Young Women." Siecus.org, accessed May 2016, http://siecus.org/index.cfm?fuseaction=Feature.showFeature&featureid=1501&pageid=518&parentid=514.

7. "Sexual Assault and the LGBT Community." HRC.org, accessed May 2016, http://www.hrc.org/resources/sexual-assault-and-the-lgbt-community.

8. "Transgender People and HIV: What We Know." HRC.org, accessed May 2016, http://www.hrc.org/resources/transgender-people-and-hiv-what-we-know.

9. "LGBT Students Experience Pervasive Harassment and Discrimination, But School-Based Resources and Supports Are Making a Difference." Glsen.org, accessed May 2016, https://www.glsen.org/article/2015-national-school-climate-survey.

10. "Lesbian, Gay, Bisexual, and Transgender Health." Glsen.org, accessed May 2016, http://www.cdc.gov/lgbthealth/youth.htm.

11. Park and Mykhyalyshyn. "L.G.B.T. People Are More Likely to Be Targets of Hate Crimes Than Any Other Minority Group." NYTimes.com, accessed June 2016, http://www.nytimes.com/interactive/2016/06/16/us/hate-crimes-against-lgbt.html?_r=1.

12. "Uniform Crime Reports." FBI.gov, accessed June 2016, https://www.fbi.gov/about-us/cjis/ucr/ucr-publications#Hate.

13. 2015 Report On Lesbian, Gay, Bisexual, Transgender, Queer and HIV-Affected Hate Violence. Anti-Violence Project, accessed June 2016, http://www.avp.org/resources/avp-resources/520-2015-report-on-lesbian-gay-bisexual-transgender-queer-and-hiv-affected-hate-violence.

14. Mona Chalabi. "Killings of LGBT and HIV-Affected People Rose 20% in 2015, Report Finds." *The Guardian*, accessed June 2016, https://www.theguardian.com/world/2016/jun/13/lgbt-hiv-killings-rose-20-percent-2015-orlando-nightclub-shooting-doubles-2016.

15. S. T. Russell and K. Joyner."Adolescent Sexual Orientation and Suicide Risk: Evidence from a National Study." *American Journal of Public Health* 91 (2001): 1276–81.

16. "Statistics About Youth Suicide." YSPP.org, accessed May 2016, http://www.yspp.org/about_suicide/statistics.htm.

17. "Suicide Facts." Suicide Prevention Education for Kids, accessed January 2016, http://www.speakforthem.org/facts.html.

# CHAPTER THIRTY-FIVE

1. Ami Kaplan. "Discussions of Mental Health Issues for Gender Variant and Transgender Individuals, Friends and Family." Transgender Mental Health, accessed July 2016, https://tgmentalhealth.com/2010/08/06/confusion-around-changing-sexual-orientation-for-trans-people.

## CHAPTER THIRTY-SIX

1. "Homophobia." AllAboutCounseling.com, accessed August 2016, http://www.allaboutcounseling.com/library/homophobia.

2. Family Acceptance Project. "Family Rejection as a Predictor of Negative Health Outcomes in White and Latino Lesbian, Gay, and Bisexual Young Adults." *Pediatrics* 123 (1), 346–52.

## CHAPTER THIRTY-SEVEN

1. "Gender Dysphoria." DSM5.org, American Psychiatric Association, accessed June 2016, http://www.dsm5.org/documents/gender%20dysphoria%20fact%20sheet.pdf.

2. Gary J. Gates. "How Many People Are Lesbian, Gay, Bisexual and Transgender?" The Williams Institute at UCLA School of Law, April 2011, accessed April 2011, http://williamsinstitute.law.ucla.edu/research/census-lgbt-demographics-studies/how-many-people-are-lesbian-gay-bisexual-and-transgender.

3. Ibid.

## CHAPTER THIRTY-EIGHT

1. "LGBTQ Youth." Centers for Disease Control and Prevention, accessed February 2017, https://www.cdc.gov/lgbthealth/youth.htm.

2. "How Do Mental Health Conditions Affect the LGBTQ Community?" National Alliance on Mental Health Issues, accessed May 2016, http://www.nami.org/Find-Support/LGBTQ.

3. "LGBTQ Youth." Centers for Disease Control and Prevention, accessed May 2016, http://www.cdc.gov/lgbthealth/youth.htmLgbtq.

4. Ibid.

## CHAPTER FORTY

1. "STUDY: 40 Percent Of Homeless Youth Are LGBT, Family Rejection Is Leading Cause." Think Progress, accessed July 2012, https://thinkprogress.org/study-40-percent-of-homeless-youth-are-lgbt-family-rejection-is-leading-cause-a2aaa72c414a#.arscdem7l.

# BIBLIOGRAPHY

Advocates for Youth. "The History of Federal Abstinence-Only Funding." http://www.advocatesforyouth.org/publications/429?task=view. Accessed July 2011.

Ahmed, Murad. "Teen 'Sexting' Craze Leading to Child Porn Arrests in U.S." *The Times* (London). https://www.thetimes.co.uk/article/teen-sexting-craze-leading-to-child-porn-arrests-in-us-2tlhkgmtqsr. Accessed January 2009.

AIDS.gov. "Preventing Sexual Transmission of HIV." https://www.hiv.gov/hiv-basics/hiv-prevention/reducing-sexual-risk/preventing-sexual-transmission-of-hiv. Accessed November 2016.

"Alice" (a team of Columbia University health educators, health care providers, other health professionals, and information and research specialists and writers). "Masturbation Healthy?" http://goaskalice.columbia.edu/answered-questions/masturbation-healthy. Accessed February 2011.

AllAboutCounseling.com. "Homophobia." https://www.allaboutcounseling.com/library/homophobia. Accessed August 2016.

American Academy of Pediatrics. "Media and Children." https://www.aap.org/en-us/advocacy-and-policy/aap-health-initiatives/pages/media-and-children.aspx. Accessed April 2014.

American College of Obstetricians and Gynecologists, Committee on Adolescent Health. "The Initial Reproductive Health Visit." *Obstetrics and Gynecology* 2010: 240–43.

American Psychiatric Association. "Gender Dysphoria." https://www.psychiatry.org/patients-families/gender-dysphoria. Accessed June 2016.

American Psychiatric Association. "Therapies Focused on Attempts to Change Sexual Orientation." http://www.psychiatry.org/File%20Library/Learn/Archives/Position-2000-Therapies-Change-Sexual-Orientation.pdf. Accessed August 2011.

# BIBLIOGRAPHY

Anti-Violence Project. "2015 Report on Lesbian, Gay, Bisexual, Transgender, Queer, and HIV-Affected Hate Violence." https://avp.org/wp-content/up loads/2017/04/ncavp_hvreport_2015_final.pdf. Accessed June 2016.

Association for Lesbian Gay, Bisexual and Transgender Issues in Counseling. "Famous LGBT People." http://www.algbtical.org/2A%20PEOPLE.htm. Accessed October 2017.

The Atlantic.com. "LGBT Students Are Not Safe At School." https://www.theatlantic.com/education/archive/2016/10/school-is-still-not-safe-for-lgbt-students/504368/. Accessed October 2017.

Bales, Kevin. "The Number." The CNN Freedom Project Ending Modern Day Slavery. http://thecnnfreedomproject.blogs.cnn.com/category/the-facts/the-number/. Accessed November 2015.

Benaroch, Roy. "Preventing Teen Suicide." WebMD.com. http://teens.webmd.com/preventing-teen-suicide#1. Accessed February 2012.

Betkowski, Bev. "Rural Teen Boys Most Likely to Access Pornography, Study Shows." Faculty News, University of Alberta. https://www.eurekalert.org/pub _releases/2007-02/uoa-oit022307.php. Accessed March 2016.

Biology News Net. "Homosexual Behavior Due to Genetics and Environmental Factors." http://www.biologynews.net/archives/2008/06/29/homosexual_behavior _due_to_genetics_and_environmental_factors.html. Accessed June 2011.

Black, Michelle. "The National Intimate Partner and Sexual Violence Survey." Centers for Disease Control and Prevention, National Center for Injury Prevention and Control, Division of Violence Prevention. http://vawnet.org/ Assoc_Files_VAWnet/NRCWebinar_NISVSBriefingHandout.pdf. Accessed December 2015.

Bogaert, Anthony. "Exactly What Percentage of the World's Population Is Asexual?" Queerty.com. http://www.queerty.com/exactly-what-percentage-of -the-worlds-population-is-asexual-20150727. Accessed July 2016.

Boonstra, Heather. "Condoms, Contraceptives and Nonoxynol-9: Complex Issues Obscured by Ideology." *Guttmacher Report on Public Policy* 8 (2) (May 2005): 4–6, 16.

Bowman, Darcia Harris. "Survey of Students Documents the Extent of Bullying." *Education Week*, May 2, 2001, http://www.edweek.org/ew/articles/2001/ 05/02/33bully.h20.html. Accessed May 2016.

Brent, Bill. *The Ultimate Guide to Anal Sex for Men* (San Francisco: Cleis Press, 2002).

British Broadcasting Corporation News. "Curtains for Semi-Nude Justice Statue." http://news.bbc.co.uk/2/hi/1788845.stm. Accessed May 2011.

Case, William. *The Art of Kissing*, Third Edition (New York: St. Martin's Griffin, 1995).

Centers for Disease Control and Prevention. "The ABCs of Viral Hepatitis." http://www.cdc.gov/Features/ViralHepatitis. Accessed August 2011.

Centers for Disease Control and Prevention. "CDC Morbidity and Mortality Weekly Report: Sexual Identity, Sex of Sexual Contacts, and Health-Related Behaviors Among Students in Grades 9–12—United States and Selected Sites, 2015." https://www.cdc.gov/mmwr/volumes/65/ss/ss6509a1.htm. Accessed August 2016.

Centers for Disease Control and Prevention. "Condoms and STDs." http://www.cdc.gov/condomeffectiveness/docs/condoms_and_stds.pdf. Accessed December 2014.

Centers for Disease Control and Prevention. "Gonorrhea—CDC Fact Sheet." http://www.cdc.gov/std/gonorrhea/stdfact-gonorrhea.htm. Accessed June 2011.

Centers for Disease Control and Prevention. "HIV Among Youth." http://www.cdc.gov/hiv/group/age/youth. Accessed July 2016.

Centers for Disease Control and Prevention. "HIV Transmission." https://www.cdc.gov/hiv/basics/prevention.html. Accessed March 2011.

Centers for Disease Control and Prevention. "Lesbian, Gay, Bisexual, and Transgender Health." http://www.cdc.gov/lgbthealth/youth.htm. Accessed May 2016.

Centers for Disease Control and Prevention. "LGBTQ Youth." http://www.cdc.gov/lgbthealth/youth.htmLgbtq. Accessed May 2016.

Centers for Disease Control and Prevention. "Reported Cases of Sexually Transmitted Diseases on the Rise, Some at Alarming Rate." https://www.cdc.gov/nchhstp/newsroom/2015/std-surveillance-report-press-release.html. Accessed November 2015.

Centers for Disease Control and Prevention. "Sexual Identity, Sex of Sexual Contacts, and Health-Risk Behaviors Among Students in Grades 9–12: Youth Risk Behavior Surveillance." https://www.researchgate.net/publication/281044134_Sexual_identity_sex_of_sexual_contacts_and_health-risk_behaviors_among_students_ in_grades_9-12-Youth_Risk_Behavior_Surveillance_selected_sites_Unites_States. Accessed June 2013.

Centers for Disease Control and Prevention. "STDs in Adolescents and Young Adults." http://www.cdc.gov/std/stats09/adol.htm. Accessed December 2010.

Centers for Disease Control and Prevention. "Syphilis & MSM (Men Who Have Sex With Men)—CDC Fact Sheet." https://www.cdc.gov/std/Syphilis/ STDFact-MSM-Syphilis.htm. Accessed April 2016.

Chalabi, Mona. "Killings of LGBT and HIV-Affected People Rose 20% in 2015, Report Finds." *The Guardian.* https://www.theguardian.com/world/2016/ jun/13/lgbt-hiv-killings-rose-20-percent-2015-orlando-nightclub-shooting -doubles-2016. Accessed June 2016.

Childress, Sarah. "CDC Reports Troubling Rise in HIV Infections Among Young People." PBS.org. http://www.pbs.org/wgbh/frontline/article/cdc-reports -troubling-rise-in-hiv-infections-among-young-people/. Accessed July 2016.

Clawson, Heather J. et al. "Human Trafficking Into and Within the United States: A Review of the Literature." Office of the Assistant Secretary for Planning and Evaluation, US Department of Health and Social Services. http:// aspe.hhs.gov/basic-report/human-trafficking-and-within-united-states-review -literature. Accessed November 2015.

Coleman E. et al. "Standards of Care for the Health of Transsexual, Transgender, and Gender-Nonconforming People." *International Journal of Transgenderism* 13 (4), 165–232. Accessed February 2016. doi:10.1080/15532739. 2011.

Cottrell, B. H. "An Updated Review of Evidence to Discourage Douching." *American Journal of Maternal Child Nursing* 35 (2) (March–April 2010): 102–7; quiz 108–9.

Cullins, Vanessa. "Chlamydia." Planned Parenthood. https://www.plannedparenthood.org/learn/stds-hiv-safer-sex/chlamydia. Accessed June 2011.

Cullins, Vanessa. "Condom." Planned Parenthood. https://www.plannedparenthood.org/learn/birth-control/condom. Accessed February 2015.

Dastagir, Alla. "The Imaginary Predator in America's Transgender Bathroom War." USAToday.com. https://www.usatoday.com/story/news/nation/2016/04/28/ transgender-bathroom-bills-discrimination/32594395/. Accessed June 2016.

Dave, S., A. M. Johnson, K. A. Fenton, C. H. Mercer, B. Erens, and K. Wellings. "Male Circumcision in Britain: Findings from a National Probability Sample Survey." *Sexually Transmitted Infections* 79 (2003): 499–500.

Davis, K. et al. "Young Men's Condom Use Resistance Tactics: A Latent Profile Analysis." *Journal of Sex Research* 51 (4): 454–65.

De Becker, Gavin. *The Gift of Fear* (New York: Dell Publishing, 1997).

Dentato, Michael. "The Minority Stress Perspective." American Psychological Association. http://www.apa.org/pi/aids/resources/exchange/2012/04/minority-stress.aspx. Accessed June 2016.

Dixon, Ejeris et al. "Hate Violence Against Lesbian, Gay, Bisexual, Transgender, Queer and HIV-Affected Communities." AVP.org. National Coalition of Anti-Violence Programs. http://avp.org/wp-content/uploads/2017/06/NCAVP_2016HateViolence_REPORT.pdf. Accessed July 2016.

DoSomething.org. "11 Facts About Teens and STIs." https://www.dosomething.org/facts/11-facts-about-teens-and-stds. Accessed June 2011.

DSM5.org./American Psychiatric Association. "Gender Dysphoria." https://www.psychiatry.org/patients-families/gender-dysphoria. Accessed June 2016.

Duggan, Maeve. "Online Harassment: Summary of Findings." Pew Research Center. http://www.pewinternet.org/2014/10/22/online-harassment/. Accessed October 2015.

Em & Lo. "The Bottom Line." *New York* Magazine. October 25, 2007.

Entertainment Software Rating Board. "ESRB Ratings Guide." http://www.esrb.org/ratings/principles_guidelines.jsp. Accessed April 2014.

Estronaut, A Forum for Women's Health. "Plan B: The New Morning After Pill." http://www.estronaut.com/a/Plan_B_Morning_After_Emergency_Contraceptive.htm. Accessed 2011.

Fagan, Patrick, and Robert Rector. "The Effects of Divorce on America." http://www.heritage.org/marriage-and-family/report/the-effects-divorce-america. Accessed July 2016.

Family Acceptance Project. "Family Rejection as a Predictor of Negative Health Outcomes in White and Latino Lesbian, Gay, and Bisexual Young Adults." *Pediatrics* 123 (1), 346–52.

Federal Bureau of Investigation. "Uniform Crime Reports." https://ucr.fbi.gov/ucr-publications#Hate. Accessed June 2016.

Finer, Lawrence. "Trends in Premarital Sex in the United States." *Public Health Reports* 122 (1) (January–February 2007): 73–78.

Flores, Andrew et al. "How Many Adults Identify as Transgender in the United States." The Williams' Institute. https://williamsinstitute.law.ucla.edu/research/how-many-adults-identify-as-transgender-in-the-united-states. Accessed July 2016.

Ford, Zack. "STUDY: 40 Percent Of Homeless Youth Are LGBT, Family Rejection Is Leading Cause." Thinkprogress.org. https://thinkprogress.org/study-40-percent-of-homeless-youth-are-lgbt-family-rejection-is-leading-cause-a2aaa72c414a. Accessed July 2016.

Frezieres, R. G. et al. "Breakage and Acceptability of a Polyurethane Condom: A Randomized, Controlled Study." https://www.ncbi.nlm.nih.gov/pubmed/9561872. Accessed February 2015.

Gardasil.com. "Information About Gardasil." https://www.gardasil9.com. Accessed August 2011.

Gates, Gary J. "How Many People Are Lesbian, Gay, Bisexual and Transgender?" The Williams Institute at UCLA School of Law. http://williamsinstitute.law.ucla.edu/research/census-lgbt-demographics-studies/how-many-people-are-lesbian-gay-bisexual-and-transgender/. Accessed April 2011.

Gay & Lesbian Alliance Against Defamation (GLAAD). "Accelerating Acceptance." http://www.glaad.org/files/2016_GLAAD_Accelerating_Acceptance.pdf. Accessed July 2017.

Gay & Lesbian Alliance Against Defamation (GLAAD). "Kevin Keller Receives Outstanding Comic Book at GLAADAwards." https://www.glaad.org/tags/dan-parent. Accessed October 2017.

Gay & Lesbian Alliance Against Defamation (GLAAD). "Tips for Allies of Transgender People." https://www.glaad.org/transgender/allies. Accessed April 2014.

Gay, Lesbian & Straight Education Network. "LGBT Students Experience Pervasive Harassment and Discrimination, But School-Based Resources and Supports Are Making a Difference." http://www.glsen.org/article/2013-national-school-climate-survey#sthash.lHXqybKM.dpuf. Accessed May 2016.

Gay, Lesbian & Straight Education Network. "Out Online: The Experiences of Gay and Lesbian, Gay, Bisexual and Transgender Youth on the Internet." https://www.glsen.org/content/out-online. Accessed October 2017.

Gay Straight Alliance Network. "10 Steps for Starting a GSA." https://gsanetwork.org/resources/building-your-gsa/10-steps-starting-gsa. Accessed August 2016.

Fields, Peter. "The Truth About Homophobia." *Huffington Post*, accessed October 2017, https://www.huffingtonpost.com/entry/the-truth-about-homophobia_us_57ae12aee4b0ae60ff026207.

Gendercentre.org. "Feminising Hormone Information." https://gendercentre.org.au/images/Services/Male_to_Female/Feminising_Hormone_Information.pdf. Accessed July 2016.

Gendercentre.org. "Masculinising Hormone Information." https://gendercentre.org.au/images/Services/Female_to_Male/Masculinising_Hormone_Information.pdf. Accessed July 2016.

Gerressu, M. et al. "Prevalence of Masturbation and Associated Factors in a British National Probability Survey." *Archives of Sexual Behavior* 37 (2) (April 2008): 266–78.

Gibbs, Jeremy. "Religious Conflict, Sexual Identity, and Suicidal Behaviors Among LGBT Young Adults." US National Library of Medicine/National Institutes of Health. https://www.ncbi.nlm.nih.gov/pubmed/25763926. Accessed June 2016.

Grant, R. M. et al.: iPrEx Study Team. "Preexposure Chemoprophylaxis for HIV Prevention in Men Who Have Sex with Men." *New England Journal of Medicine* 363 (27) (2010): 2587–99. Accessed November 2015. http://www.nejm.org/doi/full/10.1056/NEJMoa1011205#t=article.

Güntürkün, Onur. "Adult Persistence of Head-Turning Asymmetry." *Nature* (February 13, 2003), 421, 711.

HarrisInteractive. "Cyberbullying." *Trends & Tudes*, April 2007 (vol. 6, issue 4).

http://www.ncpc.org/resources/files/pdf/bullying/Cyberbullying%20Trends%20-%20Tudes.pdf.

Haeberle, Edwin. *The Sex Atlas* (New York: The Continuum Publishing Company, 1983).

Harlap, S., K. Kost, and J. D. Forrest. *Preventing Pregnancy, Protecting Health: A New Look at Birth Control Choices in the United States.* (New York: The Guttmacher Institute, 1991).

Harvard School of Public Health. "'Virginity Pledges' by Adolescents May Bias Their Reports of Premarital Sex." http://news.harvard.edu/gazette/story/2006/05/virginity-pledges-by-adolescents-may-bias-their-reports-of-premarital-sex/. Accessed June 2011.

BIBLIOGRAPHY

Hembree, Wylie C. et al. "Endocrine Treatment of Transsexual Persons: An Endocrine Society Clinical Practice Guideline." Endocrine Society. https://academic.oup.com/jcem/article/94/9/3132/2596324/Endocrine-Treatment-of-Transsexual-Persons-An. Accessed June 2016.

Henry, Shawn. "Shawn Henry on Cyber Safety." Federal Bureau of Investigation. http://www.fbi.gov/news/videos/henry_051611. Accessed April 2014.

Hepatitis B Foundation. "Hepatitis B Foundation Participates in U.S. Capitol Briefing." http://www.hepb.org/pdf/Capitol_Briefing7_05.pdf. Accessed July 2011.

Herbenick, Debby. "Erect Penile Length and Circumference Dimensions of 1,661 Sexually Active Men in the United States." *Journal of Sexual Medicine* 11 (January 2014): 93–101.

Herpes Clinic. "Genital Herpes Statistics." http://www.herpesclinic.com/genital herpes/genitalherpesstatistics/. Accessed March 2016.

Hershberger, Scott L. and Anthony R. D'Augelli. "The Impact of Victimization on the Mental Health and Suicidality of Lesbian, Gay, and Bisexual Youths." *Developmental Psychology* 31 (1), January 1995.

Huffington Post. "Study: Half of Men May Be Infected with HPV." http://www.huffingtonpost.com/2011/02/28/half-men-infected-hpv_n_829449.html. Accessed March 2011.

Human Rights Campaign. "Matthew Shepard and James Byrd, Jr. Hate Crimes Prevention Act." http://www.hrc.org/resources/hate-crimes-law. Accessed November 2011.

Human Rights Campaign. "Sexual Assault and the LGBT Community." http://www.hrc.org/resources/sexual-assault-and-the-lgbt-community. Accessed May 2016.

Human Rights Campaign. "Teen Dating Violence Among LGBTQ Youth." http://www.hrc.org/resources/teen-dating-violence-among-lgbtq-youth. Accessed July 2016.

Human Rights Campaign. "Transgender People and HIV: What We Know." http://www.hrc.org/resources/transgender-people-and-hiv-what-we-know. Accessed May 2016.

"Human Sexual Behavior." *Journal of Evolutionary Philosophy*. http://www.evolutionary-philosophy.net/human_sexuality.html. Accessed August 2011.

Hunt, Jerome. "Why the Gay and Transgender Population Experiences Higher Rates of Substance Use." Center for American Progress. https://www.american progress.org/issues/lgbt/reports/2012/03/09/11228/why-the-gay-and-transgen-der-population-experiences-higher-rates-of-substance-use/. Accessed June 2016.

Internet Crimes Against Children. "Youth Internet Safety Survey." http://www .ojp.usdoj.gov/ovc/publications/bulletins/internet_2_2001/internet_2_01_6. html. Accessed July 2011.

Johns Hopkins Medical Center, Breast Center. "Breast Self-Exams." http:// www.hopkinsmedicine.org/breast_center/treatments_services/breast_cancer_ screening/breast_self_exam.html. Accessed November 2015.

Johnson, Ramon. "Gay Population Statistics." Liveabout.com. https://www .liveabout.com/gay-population-statistics-in-the-united-states-1410784. Ac-cessed June 2016.

Kaiser Family Foundation. "STDs in America: How Many Cases and at What Cost?" http://kff.org/hivaids/sexually-transmitted-diseases-in-america-how -many. Accessed March 2016.

Kaiser Family Foundation. "U.S. Teen Sexual Activity." http://enrichmentjour-nal.ag.org/200604/200604_4USTeenSexActi.pdf. Accessed March 2016.

Kane, Jessica. "Here's How Much a Woman's Period Will Cost Her Over a Lifetime." Huffington Post. http://www.huffingtonpost.com/2015/05/18/period -cost-lifetime_n_7258780.html. Accessed October 2015.

Kaplan, Ami. "Discussions of Mental Health Issues for Gender Variant and Transgender Individuals, Friends and Family." Transgender Mental Health. https://tgmentalhealth.com/2010/08/06/confusion-around-changing-sexual-ori entation-for-trans-people/. Accessed July 2016.

Kellway, Mitch. "Blocking Puberty Is Beneficial for Transgender Youth." Ad-vocate.com. https://www.advocate.com/politics/transgender/2014/09/14/study -blocking-puberty-beneficial-transgender-youth. Accessed June 2016.

KidsHealth. "Boys and Puberty." http://kidshealth.org/kid/grow/boy/boys_pu berty.html. Accessed June 2011.

The Kinsey Institute. "Kinsey's Heterosexual-Homosexual Rating Scale." https:// www.kinseyinstitute.org/research/publications/kinsey-scale.php. Accessed Sep-tember 2011.

Klickitat County Public Health. "Abstinence." http://www.klickitatcounty.org/358/Abstinence. Accessed February 2011.

Know Your Rights. "Passports." http://www.transequality.org/know-your-rights/passports. Accessed July 2016.

Koss, Mary and Mary Harvey. *The Rape Victim: Clinical and Community Interventions* (Newbury Park, CA: Sage Library of Social Research, 1991).

Lambda Legal. "FAQ About Identity Documents." https://www.lambdalegal.org/know-your-rights/article/trans-identity-document-faq. Accessed July 2016.

Langford, Jo. *Spare Me 'The Talk!' A Guy's Guide to Sex, Relationships and Growing Up* (ParentMap, Seattle, 2015).

Langford, Jo. *Spare Me 'The Talk!' A Girl's Guide to Sex, Relationships and Growing Up* (ParentMap, Seattle, 2016).

The Leadership Conference. "Stonewall Riots: The Beginning of the LGBT Movement." http://archives.civilrights.org/archives/2009/06/449-stonewall.html. Accessed June 2016.

Lee, Carol. "Gay Teens Ignored by High School Sex Ed Classes." Women's eNews. http://womensenews.org/2002/02/gay-teens-ignored-high-school-sex-ed-classes/. Accessed December 2015.

Lowe, Franklin. "All About Semen." Menstuff. http://www.menstuff.org/issues/byissue/semen.html. Accessed July 2011.

Maltz, Wendy. *The Sexual Healing Journey: A Guide for Survivors of Sexual Abuse.* (New York: HarperCollins, 2001), 30.

Masters, William H. and Virginia Johnson. *Human Sexual Response* (New York: Bantam, 1981).

The Mayo Clinic. "Toxic Shock Syndrome." http://www.mayoclinic.org/diseases-conditions/toxic-shock-syndrome/home/ovc-20317877. Accessed October 2015.

McCullom, Rod. "Lowering the Age for HIV Prevention." *The Atlantic.* https://www.theatlantic.com/health/archive/2015/02/lowering-the-age-for-hiv-prevention/385303/. Accessed November 2015.

McDermon, Brendan. The Power of Inclusive Sex-Ed. *The Atlantic,* accessed October 2017, https://www.theatlantic.com/education/archive/2017/07/the-power-of-inclusive-sex-ed/533772/.

McKeon, Brigid. "Effective Sex Education." Advocates for Youth. http://www.advocatesforyouth.org/publications/450?task=view. Accessed October 2011.

The Medical Center for Female Sexuality. "Female Orgasm." http://www.centerforfemalesexuality.com/orgasm.html. Accessed April 2011.

Medical News Today. "Increase in Anal Intercourse Involving At-risk Teens and Young Adults." http://www.medicalnewstoday.com/releases/130181.php. Accessed January 2011.

Merck and Co. Inc. "Hepatitis B Vaccine (Recombinant)." https://www.merckvaccines.com/Products/RecombivaxHB/Pages/home. Accessed July 2011.

Meyer, Ilan. "Prejudice, Social Stress, and Mental Health in Lesbian, Gay, and Bisexual Populations: Conceptual Issues and Research Evidence." National Institutes of Health. http://www.ncbi.nlm.nih.gov/pmc/articles/PMC2072932. Accessed June 2016.

Meyer, Ilan and Mary Northridge. *The Health of Sexual Minorities: Public Health Perspectives on Lesbian, Gay, Bisexual and Transgender Populations* (New York: Springer, 2007).

Minnesota Department of Health. "STD Awareness Month Facts." http://www.health.state.mn.us/divs/idepc/dtopics/stds/stdbasics.html. Accessed April 2011.

Morris, Jessica F., Craig R. Waldo, and Esther D. Rothblum. "A Model of Predictors and Outcomes of Outness Among Lesbian and Bisexual Women." *American Journal of Orthopsychiatry, Mental Health and Social Justice.* https://www.ncbi.nlm.nih.gov/pubmed/11271718. Accessed May 2016.

My Internet Safety Coach. "Online Safety Statistics." http://myinternetsafetycoach.com/?p=18. Accessed December 2010.

National Alliance on Mental Health Issues. "How Do Mental Health Conditions Affect the LGBTQ Community?" http://www.nami.org/Find-Support/LGBTQ. Accessed May 2016.

The National Breast Cancer Foundation. "Symptoms and Signs." http://www.nationalbreastcancer.org/breast-cancer-symptoms-and-signs. Accessed November.

The National Campaign to Prevent Teen and Unplanned Pregnancy. "*Sex and Tech: Results from a Survey of Teens and Young Adults.*" http://thenationalcampaign.org/resource/sex-and-tech. Accessed December 2014.

National Center for Missing and Exploited Children. "Key Facts." http://www
.missingkids.com/KeyFacts. Accessed August 2015.

National Center for Missing and Exploited Children. "Teen Online and Wireless Safety Survey: Cyberbullying, Sexting and Parental Controls." http://
www.cox.com/wcm/en/aboutus/datasheet/takecharge/2009-teen-survey.pdf.
Accessed May 2016.

The National Center for Victims of Crime. "Child Sexual Abuse Statistics."
http://victimsofcrime.org/media/reporting-on-child-sexual-abuse/child-sexual
-abuse-statistics. Accessed November 2016.

National Institutes of Health. "Pelvic Floor Anatomy and Applied Physiology."
https://www.ncbi.nlm.nih.gov/pmc/articles/PMC2617789/. Accessed October
2017.

National Institutes of Health/US National Library of Medicine. "Your Guide
to Understanding Genetic Conditions." https://ghr.nlm.nih.gov/chromosome/
Y. Accessed May 2016.

National Victim Center. "Factsheets: Teen Dating Violence." http://www
.svfreenyc.org/survivors_factsheet_48.html. Accessed November 2015.

News Medical Life Sciences. "1,500 Animal Species Practice Homosexuality."
http://www.news-medical.net/news/2006/10/23/1500-animal-species-practice
-homosexuality.aspx. Accessed September 2016.

New York State Department of Health. "Gonorrhea Gonococcal Infection."
https://www.health.ny.gov/diseases/communicable/gonorrhea/fact_sheet.htm
. Accessed November 2010.

Nivin, Todd. "Menstrual Blood Problems." WebMD. http://www.webmd.com/
women/guide/normal-period. Accessed October 2015.

"Out Magazine's Power 50 2017." Out Magazine. https://www.out.com/
power-50/2017/7/19/power-50-2017. Accessed October 2017.

Parents and Friends of Lesbians and Gays (PFLAG). "Be Yourself: Questions
and Answers for Gay, Lesbian and Bisexual Youth." http://seattle-pflag.org/
pflag/wp-content/uploads/2015/03/Be-Yourself.pdf. Accessed March 2016.

Parents and Friends of Lesbians and Gays (PFLAG). "Statistics You Should
Know About Gay & Transgender Students." http://www.pflagnyc.org/safe
schools/statistics. Accessed June 2016.

Park, Haeyoun and Iaryna Mykhyalshyn. "L.G.B.T. People Are More Likely To Be Targets of Hate Crimes Than Any Other Minority Group." nytimes.com. http://www.nytimes.com/interactive/2016/06/16/us/hate-crimes-against-lgbt .html?_r=1NYTimes.com. Accessed June 2016.

Pereira, Rodrigues. "Internalized Homophobia and Suicidal ideation Among LGBT Youth." *Journal of Psychiatry*. https://www.omicsonline.org/open-access/ internalized-homophobia-and-suicidal-ideation-among-lgb-youth-Psychia-try-1000229.php?aid=41252. Accessed June 2016.

Pew Research Center. "Small Share of Americans in Active Military Duty." http://www.pewresearch.org/fact-tank/2012/05/23/small-share-of-americans -in-active-military-duty/. Accessed July 2016.

Pew Research Center. "A Survey of LGBT Americans." http://www.pewsocial-trends.org/2013/06/13/a-survey-of-lgbt-americans. Accessed June 2016.

Pew Research Center. "Teens, Kindness and Cruelty on Social Network Sites." http://www.pewinternet.org/2011/11/09/teens-kindness-and-cruelty-on-social -network-sites-2. Accessed November 2011.

Planned Parenthood. "Comparing Effectiveness of Birth Control Methods." https://www.plannedparenthood.org/learn/birth-control. Accessed December 2010.

Planned Parenthood. "Puberty." https://www.plannedparenthood.org/learn/ teens/puberty. Accessed February 2015.

Planned Parenthood. "Sexually Transmitted Diseases (STDs)." https://www .plannedparenthood.org/planned-parenthood-northern-new-england/health-services/sexually-transmitted-infections-stis. Accessed June 2011.

Potok, Mark. "Anti-Gay Hate Crimes: Doing The Math." SPLawCenter. org. https://www.splcenter.org/fighting-hate/intelligence-report/2011/anti-gay -hate-crimes-doing-math. Accessed July 2017.

Raine, T. R. et al. "One-Year Contraceptive Continuation and Pregnancy in Adolescent Girls and Women Initiating Hormonal Contraceptives." *Obstetrics & Gynecology* 117 (February 2011): 363–71. http://www.ncbi.nlm.nih.gov/ pubmed/21252751. Accessed February 2015.

RAINN.org. "Statistics." https://rainn.org/statistics. Accessed March 2016.

Remafedi, Gary, James A. Farrow, and Robert W. Deisher. "Risk Factors for Attempted Suicide in Gay and Bisexual Youth." *Pediatrics* 87 (1991): 869–75.

Reuters. "Breast Implants Linked with Suicide." http://www.reuters.com/article/us-implants-suicide-idUSN0836919020070809. Accessed November 2015.

RevelandRiot.com. "Information on Transitioning and Transgender Health." http://www.revelandriot.com/resources/trans-health/. Accessed June 2016.

Robinson, B. A. "Major U.S. Laws Concerning Abortion." Religious Tolerance. http://www.religioustolerance.org/abo_supr.htm. Accessed January 2011.

Robinson, B. A. "Reparative Therapy: Statements by Professional Associations and Their Leaders." Religious Tolerance. http://religioustolerance.org/hom_prof3.html. Accessed June 2011.

Ropelato, Jerry. "Internet Pornography Statistics." Top Ten Reviews. http://www.toptenreviews.com/internet-pornography-statistics. Accessed August 2011.

Russell, T. and K. Joyner. "Adolescent Sexual Orientation and Suicide Risk: Evidence from a National Study." *American Journal of Public Health* 2001 (91):1276–81. https://www.ncbi.nlm.nih.gov/pubmed/11499118. Accessed June 2016.

SafetyServe.com. "Get Defensive About It!" http://www.safetyserve.com/FineSource/elearning/courses/titles/NYDMVII/Session_Summary_One.pdf. Accessed January 2017.

Saletan, William. "Ass Backwards: The Media's Silence About Rampant Anal Sex." Slate. http://www.slate.com/articles/health_and_science/human_nature/2005/09/ass_backwards.html. Accessed September 2015.

Savage, Dan. "Savage Love: Play with Her Clit." *The Stranger.* July 19, 2007.

Savage, Dan. "Savage Love: Saddlebacked!" *The Stranger.* January 29, 2009.

Savage, Dan. "Savage Love: Wiggle Room." *The Stranger.* February 25, 2010.

SexLaws.org. "Sexual Offenses: Federal Law 18 U.S.C. 1466A—Obscene Visual Representations of the Sexual Abuse of Children." https://www.law.cornell.edu/uscode/text/18/1466A. Accessed March 2016.

Shapiro, Lila. "New Report Offers a Look at 'Survival Sex' and the LGBTQ Youth Who Are Turning To It." Huffington Post. http://www.slate.com/articles/health_and_science/human_nature/2005/09/ass_backwards.html. Accessed June 2016.

Siecus.org. "New Study Finds HIV Risk Among Sexual-Minority Young Women." http://siecus.org/index.cfm?fuseaction=Feature.showFeature&featurei d=1501&pageid=518&parentid=514. Accessed May 2016.

Simon, Harvey, MD. "Hepatitis B." *New York Times*. http://health.nytimes.com/ health/guides/disease/rubella/hepatitis-b.html. Accessed September 2011.

Snyder, Howard. "Sexual Assault of Young Children as Reported to Law Enforcement: Victim, Incident, and Offender Characteristics: Table 1: Age Profile of the Victims of Sexual Assault." US Department of Justice, Bureau of Justice Statistics. https://www.bjs.gov/content/pub/pdf/saycrle.pdf. Accessed December 2015.

Songhai, Barcligt. "Premenstrual Syndrome (PMS) Fact Sheet." Office of Women's Health. http://www.womenshealth.gov/publications/our-publications/ fact-sheet/premenstrual-syndrome.html. Accessed July 2011.

Spack, Norman P. et al. "Children and Adolescents with Gender Identity Disorder Referred to a Pediatric Medical Center". *Journal of Pediatrics*. http://pediat rics.aappublications.org/content/129/3/418. Accessed March 2016.

Spitzer, R. L. "The Diagnostic Status of Homosexuality in DSM-III: A Reformulation of the Issues." *American Journal of Psychiatry* 138 (1981): 210–15.

StopHomophobia.com. "Stonewall: Freedom Overdue." http://www.stop-ho mophobia.com/thestonewallriots.htm. Accessed June 2016.

Suicide Prevention Education for Kids. "Suicide Facts." http://www.speak forthem.org/facts.html. Accessed January 2016.

Tedeschi, Sara K. et al. "Vaccination in Juvenile Correctional Facilities: State Practices, Hepatitis B, and the Impact on Anticipated Sexually Transmitted Infection Vaccines." *Public Health Reports* 122 (1) (January–February 2007): 44–48.

Think Progress. "STUDY: 40 Percent Of Homeless Youth Are LGBT, Family Rejection Is Leading Cause." July 2012. https://thinkprogress.org/study-40 -percent-of-homeless-youth-are-lgbt-family-rejection-is-leading-cause-a2aaa 72c414a#.arscdem7l. Accessed July 2016.

TransgenderLawCenter.org. "Social Security Administration Updates Gender Change Policy." http://transgenderlawcenter.org/archives/8339. Accessed June 2016.

Trenholm, Christopher et al. "Impacts of Four Title V, Section 510 Abstinence Education Programs." Mathematica Policy Research Inc. http://www.mathe matica-mpr.com/publications/pdfs/impactabstinence.pdf. Accessed April 2011.

# BIBLIOGRAPHY

Truvada.com. http://www.truvada.com. Accessed December 2014.

University of Maryland, A. James Clark School of Engineering. "Study Finds Female-Name Chat Users Get 25 Times More Malicious Messages." http://ece .umd.edu/news/news_story.php?id=1788. Accessed November 2015.

US Department of Justice. "Internet Crimes Against Children." https://ojp.gov/ovc/ publications/bulletins/internet_2_2001/internet_2_01_6.html. Accessed July 2016.

TabooJive. "Stonewall: Freedom Overdue." Stop-Homophobia.com, accessed June 2016, http://www.stop-homophobia.com/thestonewallriots.htm.

US Department of Justice. "U.S. Departments of Justice and Education Release Joint Guidance to Help Schools Ensure the Civil Rights of Transgender Students." https://www.justice.gov/opa/pr/us-departments-justice-and-education-release-joint-guidance-help-schools-ensure-civil-rights. Accessed May 2016.

US Department of State. "Gender Transition Applicants." https://travel.state.gov/ content/passports/en/passports/information/gender.html. Accessed July 2016.

US National Library of Medicine. "Phthalates." https://toxtown.nlm.nih.gov/ text_version/chemicals.php?id=24. Accessed November 2015.

Van Dam, Carla. *Identifying Child Molesters* (New York: Haworth Maltreatment and Trauma Press, 2001), 50.

Van Geel, Mitch et al. "Relationship Between Peer Victimization, Cyberbullying, and Suicide in Children and Adolescents: A Meta-Analysis." *JAMA Pediatrics* 168 (5): 435–42. Published online March 10, 2014. http://www.ncbi.nlm .nih.gov/pubmed/24615300.

Veale, David, Sarah Miles, Sally Bramley, Gordon Muir, and John Hodsoll. "Am I Normal? A Systematic Review and Construction of Nomograms for Flaccid and Erect Penis Length and Circumference in Up to 15,521 Men." BJU International. Wiley Online Library. http://onlinelibrary.wiley.com/doi/10.1111/ bju.13010/full. Accessed September 2015.

Warner, Jennifer. "Premarital Sex the Norm in America." WebMD. http:// www.webmd.com/sex-relationships/news/20061220/premarital-sex-the-norm -in-america. Accessed March 2011.

WebMD. "How The Penis Works." https://www.webmd.com/erectile-dysfunc tion/how-an-erection-occurs. Accessed October 2017.

Weiss, Susan. "Date Rape Drugs Fact Sheet." Department of Health and Human Services Office on Women's Health. https://www.womenshealth.gov/a-z-topics/date-rape-drugs. Accessed August 2011.

Whedon, Joss. "Doppelgangland." *Buffy The Vampire Slayer.* Fox Television. 1999.

The Williams Institute. "Safe at School: Addressing the School Environment and LGBT Safety through Policy and Legislation." https://williamsinstitute.law.ucla.edu/research/safe-schools-and-youth/safe-at-school-addressing-the-school-environment-and-lgbt-safety-through-policy-and-legislation-2/. Accessed October 2017.

World Professional Association for Transgender Health. "Standards of Care for the Health of Transsexual, Transgender, and Gender Nonconforming People, Seventh Version (PDF)." http://www.wpath.org/site_page.cfm?pk_association _webpage_menu=1351&pk_association_webpage=3926. Accessed July 2016.

Ybarra, Michele et al. "National Rates of Adolescent Physical, Psychological, and Sexual Teen-Dating Violence." American Psychological Association. https://www.apa.org/news/press/releases/2013/08/sexual-teen.pdf. Accessed November 2015.

Youth Suicide Prevention Program. "Statistics About Youth Suicide." http://www.yspp.org/about_suicide/statistics.htm. Accessed May 2016.

Zernike, Kate. "Use of Contraception Drops, Slowing Decline of Abortion Rate." *New York Times,* May 5, 2006. http://www.nytimes.com/2006/05/05/health/05abort.html. Accessed May 2011.

Zibners, A., B. A. Cromer, and J. Hayes. "Comparison of Continuation Rates for Hormonal Contraception Among Adolescents." *Journal of Pediatric and Adolescent Gynecology* 12 (1999): 90–94. https://www.ncbi.nlm.nih.gov/pubmed/10326194.

Zimmerman, Mike. "15 Facts You Didn't Know About Your Penis." *Men's Health.* http://www.menshealth.com/sex-women/15-facts-you-didnt-know-about-your -penis. Accessed July 2011.

# INDEX

# ABOUT THE AUTHOR

**Jo Langford** is a parent, sex educator, and master-level therapist who has worked for two decades with youth in high schools, and residential, medical, and psychiatric settings.

Jo uses information, education, and humor to help families increase their knowledge and self-confidence as a proactive defense against the unfortunate consequences that sometimes accompany teen sexual behavior.

He has spent the past twenty years in private practice, centered on that intersection of youth, sexuality, technology, and behavior, providing therapy to adolescents around a range of sexuality issues as well as comprehensive sexuality education for teens and their families.

He is also an international speaker and the author of the *Spare Me 'The Talk!'* series—guides to sex, relationships, and growing up for modern teens and their parents.